10 IN 20

DR. FUHRMAN'S
LOSE 10 POUNDS IN 20 DAYS DETOX PROGRAM

Joel Fuhrman, M.D.

Published by:
Gift of Health Press

FOREWORD

I'm proud to offer you the opportunity to lose weight and, most importantly, feel better than you have in years! Losing weight fast, if done healthfully, is NOT unhealthy or a hindrance to permanent dietary improvements. It can be the healthiest thing you have ever done in your life, and spur you on to continue to eat healthfully and maintain the benefits.

I would never encourage anyone to try to lose weight fast using some gimmick or fad. Losing weight temporarily, with a program you are not going to maintain, offers no lasting benefit.

I want you to undergo a health transformation that adds a bounce to your step and makes your skin glow. Hopefully, the effortless weight loss and how great you will feel will encourage and motivate you to continue eating healthfully for the rest of your life.

I recognize that eating this healthfully can be tough for some people to maintain. But keep in mind, it is only hard at the beginning, when you are feeling poorly and detoxing from the unhealthy Standard American Diet (SAD), which I also call the DAD (Deadly American Diet). Within four to five days, you will be feeling better than ever, and watching the weight melt away as you flood your body with anti-cancer nutrients.

I know you can do it!

Wishing you the best of health always,

Joel Fuhrman

The menus and shopping lists in this booklet have been created for a single person following the **10 in 20 Detox Program**. Some of the recipes, particularly those for soups, stews and salad dressings, make multiple servings. These extra servings can be used for future meals and will help you cut down on your cooking time.

TABLE OF CONTENTS

CONNECTIONS

Sometimes, it may feel like you're the only one eating salad in a cookie-obsessed world, but you're not!

By purchasing the program, you'll be able to join the private **10 in 20 Detox Facebook page,** where you can interact with others following the 10 in 20 Detox. Its a great place to share tips, trade recipes and get inspired! Join now: www.facebook.com/groups/DrFuhrman10in20/

SHOPPING GUIDE

The ingredients for all of the recipes in this plan are available at your favorite food markets. But it can sometimes be a challenge to find prepared foods, such as salad dressings, soups and condiments, that are made without added salt, sugar, oils and starches. You'll find these products, as well as multivitamins, supplements, books, and media in our shop at **DrFuhrman.com.**

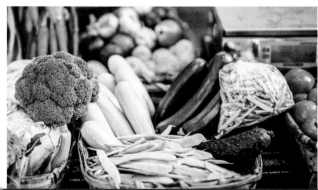

TESTIMONIAL

Allison V. followed the 10 in 20 Detox Program for 20 days, and loved the way it made her feel energized and happy. Most importantly, she lost 10 pounds without feeling hungry! She was so happy that she decided to repeat the program. After another 20 days following Dr. Fuhrman's eating style, Allison had lost a total of 16 pounds, and dropped two sizes in her clothing.

"I did have to buy new pants," she said with a laugh. "And that was a great feeling."

Allison found that following Dr. Fuhrman's plan was very rewarding, both mentally and physically.

"I'm so happy to know that I can resist unhealthy foods," she said. "And having my energy level rise, feeling lighter and clearer, and overall healthier, has been amazing. Thank you, Dr. Fuhrman!"

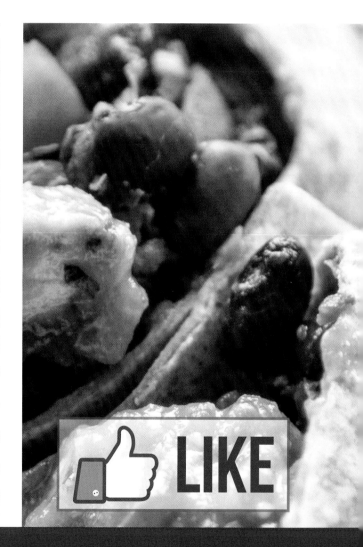

LET'S FACE IT
TRADITIONAL DIETS DON'T WORK.

Think about it. If traditional diets really worked, then everyone would be able to achieve their ideal weight with a little willpower and a commitment to laying off the "bad" foods. If traditional diets really worked, you would only have to follow them once, because there would be no danger of "yo-yo-ing" or regaining the weight. Finally, if traditional diets really worked, you would not only lose excess weight—you'd also see improvements in your overall health, and lessen your risk of serious disease.

No matter what popular diet you choose—calorie restriction, high protein, low carb, low fat, Paleo, Atkins, Zone, South Beach, Mediterranean, or many others—the results follow a predictable pattern. You start enthusiastically, determined to stick to it, no matter how hard it is. You spend your days hungry, irritable, and tormented by thoughts of "forbidden" foods. You feel rundown. And then your willpower slips—just a little at first, then some more—and then all bets are off, and you're back to where you started.

If this sounds familiar, then you're reading the right information because:

DR. FUHRMAN'S 10 IN 20 DETOX PROGRAM IS NOT A DIET. IT IS A LIFESTYLE PLAN.

Why is this plan different? The fundamental goal is to not only lose weight, but to maximize health. As a physician who always looks at the most current research, I have designed a program that supplies your body with the nutrition, micronutrients and phytochemicals it needs to achieve optimal weight and prevent disease.

A diet-style that is rich in micronutrients also suppresses your appetite and reduces food cravings!

HOW THIS "KICK START" PHASE WILL WORK

This diet is specially designed to help you drop up to 10 pounds in just 20 days. This targeted program focuses on filling your daily diet with nutrient-dense foods that will help your body use your body fat for energy, while repairing and rejuvenating valuable tissue. Following this eating style will also reset your palate, and allow you to savor the flavors of natural food.

WHAT YOU CAN EXPECT

This diet takes the guesswork out of what to eat—not only to lose weight and feel great, but also to help you overcome your cravings for toxic and unhealthy foods.

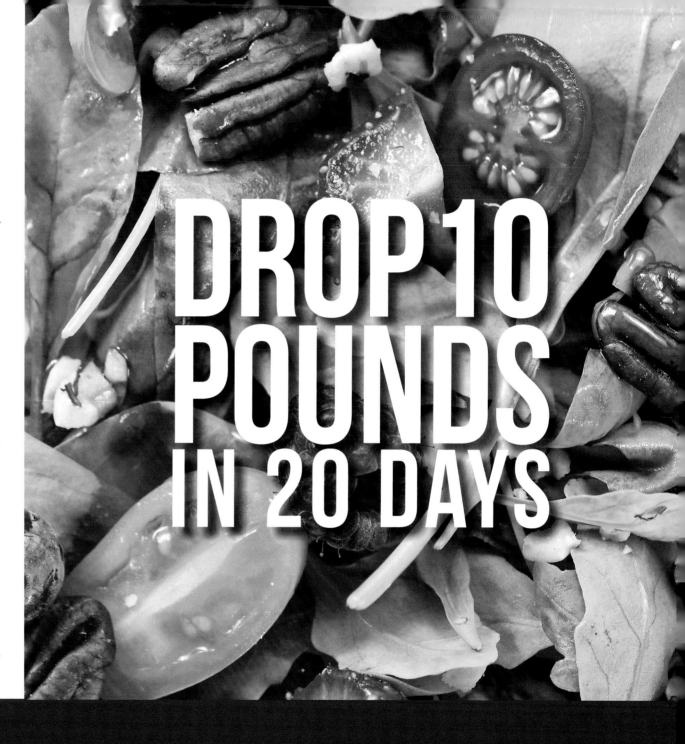

DROP 10 POUNDS IN 20 DAYS

This is not a fad diet that leaves you eating grapefruit and pickles for a week–this is a diet of body-healing, whole plant foods that is based on the latest advances in nutritional science. And, in case I forgot to mention it: The 10 in 20 program was developed to be delicious, too.

DETOXING FROM UNHEALTHY FOODS

During the first few days of this program, you may feel tired and weak; you may find yourself craving the excess salt and sugar that is no longer in your diet. This is normal. It is your body's way of detoxing from unhealthy foods. After the first three days, withdrawal symptoms from unhealthy eating habits lessen considerably. You won't be uncomfortably hungry, even with the lesser amount of calories.

WHAT'S THE CATCH?

There really isn't one, unless you'd rather hold on to those 10 extra pounds. This program will introduce you to a new way of eating, and re-introduce your palate to a world of natural textures and flavors that aren't muddied by added salt, sugar, oil and white flour.

MEET JOEL FUHRMAN, M.D.

Joel Fuhrman, M.D. is a board-certified family physician, six-time *New York Times* best-selling author, and nutritional researcher who specializes in preventing and reversing disease through nutritional and natural methods. Dr. Fuhrman is the President of the Nutritional Research Foundation. His work and discoveries are published in medical journals, and he is involved with multiple nutritional studies with major research institutions across America.

Dr. Fuhrman's the Eat to Live Retreat is a year-round residential facility located about 30 minutes from downtown San Diego, California (www.drfuhrman. com/etlretreat). Guests stay for sessions lasting 1 – 3 months. Under Dr. Fuhrman's medical care, you are immersed in the Nutritarian lifestyle, dine on organic food, attend group therapy, and learn cooking and other skills to maintain a healthy lifestyle. Your health will be transformed as you recover from diabetes, heart disease, autoimmune disease or other serious conditions as well as shed unwanted pounds. You will go home with the knowledge and strategies to continue your journey to a healthy, long and vibrant life.

Dr. Fuhrman has appeared on hundreds of radio and television shows. Through his own hugely successful PBS specials, which have raised more than $30 million for public broadcasting stations, he has brought nutritional science to homes across America and around the world. Dr. Fuhrman is the author of six *New York Times* best-sellers: *Eat to Live* (Little Brown, 2003; updated, 2011); *Super Immunity* (HarperOne, 2012); *The End of Diabetes* (HarperOne, 2013); *The Eat to Live Cookbook* (HarperOne, 2013); *The End of Dieting* (HarperOne, 2014) and *The End of Heart Disease* (HarperOne, 2016). To date, he has sold more than three million books.

In 2017, Dr. Fuhrman released *Fast Food Genocide* (HarperOne 2017), an examination of how fast food is destroying the physical, mental and emotional health of our society – and what we can do about it. He also introduced legions of food lovers to the joys of Nutritarian cooking with his *Eat to Live Quick and Easy Cookbook* (HarperOne, 2017).

Dr. Fuhrman has written several other popular books on nutritional science, which include: *Eat for Health, Disease-Proof Your Child, Fasting and Eating for Health*.

Dr. Fuhrman's new book, *Eat for Life* is his most comprehensive work, published by HarperOne in early 2020.

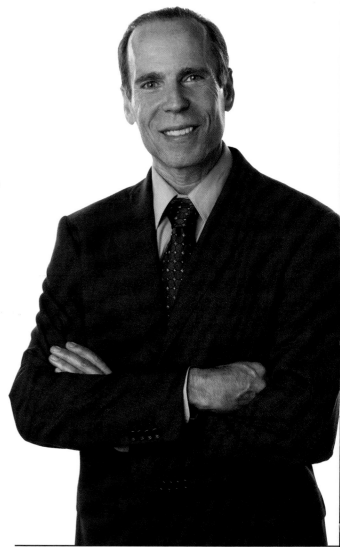

JOEL FUHRMAN, M.D.
Family Physician & Nutritional Researcher

NUTRITION AND NATURAL HEALING

WHY THE NUTRITARIAN DIET WORKS

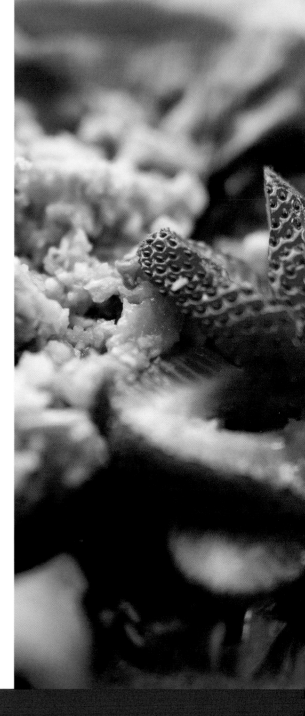

I developed the Nutritarian eating style to harness the body's tremendous power to heal itself through proper nutrition. Rooted in scientific fact rather than the latest trendy diet theories, the Nutritarian program has helped tens of thousands of people achieve sustainable weight loss, reverse chronic illnesses, and enjoy enhanced longevity.

This program is nutrient-dense and plant-rich, utilizing anti-cancer superfoods that also facilitate weight loss. These foods supply essential macronutrients (protein, carbohydrates and fat), and also provide vital micronutrients (vitamins, phytochemicals and minerals). They provide what your body needs to maximize its self-healing and self-repairing mechanisms.

Numerous diet plans call for counting calories, eliminating some foods and adding others, but only this eating style asks you to strive for more micronutrients in your diet. My recommendations are based on consuming larger quantities of nutrient-rich foods, and fewer foods with low nutritional value. As you eat more and more nutrient-dense, unprocessed foods, your appetite for empty-calorie foods decreases and you gradually lose your addiction to them. As the micronutrient quality of your diet increases, your desire to overeat is curtailed.

The most important cornerstone of health is nutrition. Without superior nutrition, your ability to live life to the fullest is limited. Consuming a low-nutrient diet

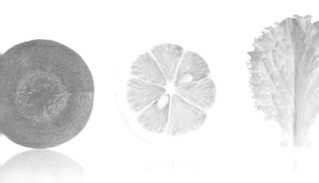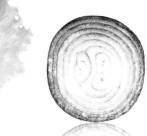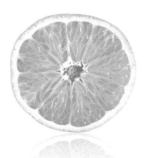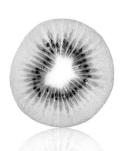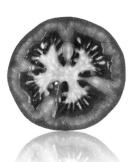

made up of empty-calorie, processed, refined foods, as well as high-fat, low-fiber animal products, greatly increases the chances that you will be overweight or obese. It also leads to a higher likelihood of developing diabetes, heart disease or cancer.

Don't assume that good health and ideal weight are the result of genetics or luck. The reality is that most of us bear the responsibility for our health and appearance through our dietary choices.

ON THIS NUTRITARIAN DIET PLAN, YOU WILL:

- Eat mainly nutrient-dense, whole plant foods: vegetables, fruit, beans, nuts, and seeds
- Eat only a small amount of animal products (these can be omitted if you prefer)
- Eliminate foods that are completely empty of nutrients such as sugar, sweeteners, white flour and processed foods

BENEFITS:

- **LOSE WEIGHT—OFTEN UP TO 10 POUNDS IN 20 DAYS**

- **LEARN NEW EATING HABITS AND TASTE PREFERENCES THAT WILL ALLOW YOU TO REACH AND MAINTAIN YOUR IDEAL BODY WEIGHT**

- **FEEL YOUR ENERGY LEVEL SOAR AS YOU DETOX FROM UNHEALTHFUL, ADDICTIVE FOODS**

- **REVERSE HIGH BLOOD PRESSURE, HIGH CHOLESTEROL, HEADACHES, INDIGESTION, ACNE, ASTHMA AND CHRONIC FATIGUE SYNDROME**

- **PROTECT YOURSELF AGAINST HEART DISEASE, STROKE, DEMENTIA, OSTEOPOROSIS AND CANCER**

THE 10 BEST FOODS

You've heard people talk about "eating the rainbow," and it's great advice. Colorful plant foods aren't just beautiful to look at—the phytochemicals, carotenoids, flavonoids and other micronutrients that give them their gorgeous hues will make your body glow with health. Here are my top ten picks for the best foods on earth.

GREEN LEAFY VEGETABLES
These foods pack a micronutrient punch. This category includes dark lettuces, kale, collard greens, arugula, and watercress.

NON-LEAFY CRUCIFEROUS VEGETABLES
Broccoli, cauliflower, Brussels sprouts and cabbage contain phytochemicals that modify hormones, detoxify compounds and prevent toxins from damaging DNA.

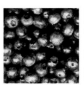

BERRIES
These fruits support heart health, improve blood glucose levels and reduce inflammation. Enjoy all berries including: blueberries, raspberries, strawberries and blackberries.

BEANS
Satisfying and versatile, beans and legumes contain high levels of soluble and insoluble fiber and resistant starch.

MUSHROOMS
White button, Portobello, shiitake, oyster and other varieties support immune function and protect against breast cancer.

ONIONS

They might make your eyes water, but onions supply anti-cancer, anti-inflammatory, and antioxidant compounds.

NUTS

Walnuts, pistachios, pine nuts and almonds protect cardiovascular health and are rich in sterols, stanols, fiber, and minerals.

SEEDS

Flax, chia, hemp, sesame, sunflower and pumpkin seeds provide all of the advantages of nuts, plus they supply omega-3 fats and anti-cancer lignans.

TOMATOES

High in the carotenoid lycopene, tomatoes have strong antioxidant and anti-inflammatory properties.

POMEGRANATES AND CHERRIES

These fruits protect against heart disease, cancer and cognitive impairment, and reduce oxidative stress.

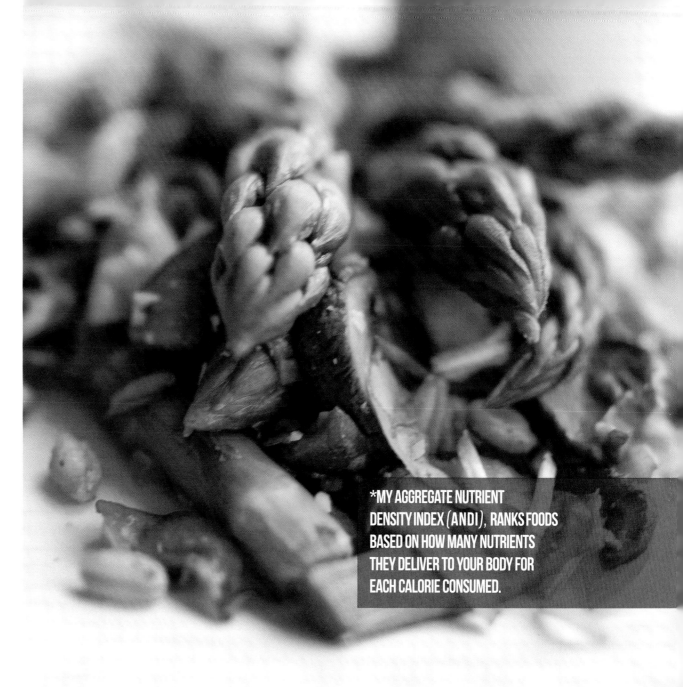

*MY AGGREGATE NUTRIENT DENSITY INDEX (ANDI), RANKS FOODS BASED ON HOW MANY NUTRIENTS THEY DELIVER TO YOUR BODY FOR EACH CALORIE CONSUMED.

FREQUENTLY ASKED QUESTIONS

Q **WILL I GET ENOUGH PROTEIN ON THE 10 IN 20 DETOX PROGRAM?**

Don't worry, you will get enough protein. The menus exceed the recommended daily value for protein.

Many so-called diet "experts" and even many doctors tell us that we need to eat large amounts of animal protein in order to stay healthy. It's a comforting story, because many people want to keep eating meat, eggs and dairy. But the truth is, plant foods contain the full spectrum of amino acids, and provide all of the protein our bodies need. Eating large amounts of animal products is not a healthy way to meet our nutritional needs.

One of the problems associated with eating animal protein is that it elevates insulin-like growth factor 1 (IGF-1) more than plant protein. That's because animal protein is richer in essential amino acids.

These elevated IGF-1 levels increase your risk of developing cardiovascular disease and cancer.

Q **IS THIS PROGRAM VEGAN?**

Animal products may be used occasionally in small amounts: 1 to 2 ounces per serving. Don't think of meat as the main course— use it as more of a flavoring or condiment. Vegan options are given for any recipe that contains an animal product.

WHAT IF I SLIP UP AND HAVE A DAY WHERE I DON'T FOLLOW THE PLAN?

Just pick up where you left off. The only failure is to stop trying.

IS IT TRUE THAT BREAKING MY FOOD INTAKE UP INTO SMALLER MEALS EATEN THROUGHOUT THE DAY IS HELPFUL?

No—you don't want to be eating throughout the day, because your body will always be in the anabolic phase (digesting) and won't go into the catabolic phase, where fat is burned for fuel and when your body is working to clean itself. Eating constantly interferes with body-fat loss, even from the same amount of caloric intake.

WHAT BEVERAGES CAN I HAVE?

Water is always the best choice for a beverage. It is okay to have plain, unsweetened seltzer or carbonated water. Hot or iced caffeine-free herbal tea is also an option.

CAN I DRINK COFFEE?

Cut out the caffeine or limit yourself to one cup of coffee per day. Coffee can be an addictive substance and it is better to consume it only in moderation, if at all. Any sweetened milk, whether dairy or non-dairy, added to the cup of coffee will hinder the full potential of this plan.

CAN I ADD SPICES OR OTHER SEASONINGS TO THE RECIPES?

Feel free to spice up your meals. You can add herbs, spices, no-salt seasonings, cayenne pepper or hot pepper flakes to any of the recipes. Just don't use salt.

HOW DO I HANDLE EATING OUT AT A RESTAURANT?

Dining out can be challenging when transitioning to a high-nutrient diet. Do some research ahead of time and look for restaurants that have healthful options. For breakfast, it is easy to find oatmeal and fresh fruit. For lunch and dinner, large, entrée-sized salads are often good choices; ask for the dressing on the side and use a minimal amount, or stick to lemon juice or vinegar. Vegetable-filled whole grain wraps or vegetable burgers are also commonly available. Most restaurants will also be happy to make you a special platter composed of an assortment of cooked vegetables.

WHAT IF I GET INVITED TO A PARTY?

Bring your own food to the party and bring extra to share with others. It is also helpful to eat something healthful before you go, so you don't arrive at the party hungry and tempted to overindulge.

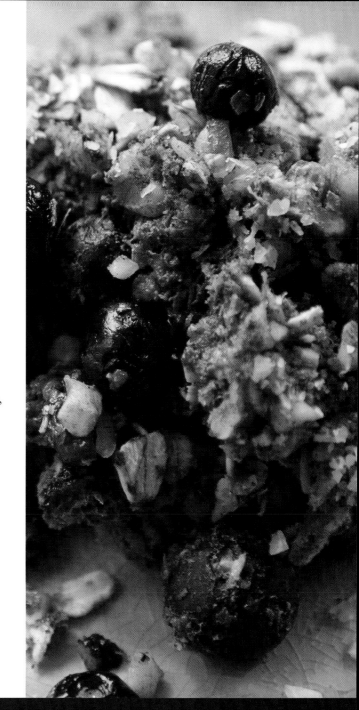

DAILY AFFIRMATIONS

Embarking on a 20-day program to lose weight and improve your health is a commitment to take care of your most prized possession: the body you were born with. Whether you have a hundred pounds to lose or are just struggling to drop those last few inches, the 10 in 20 Detox Program will put you on the right path to achieving your goals.

As you nourish your body with healing, whole foods —and stop eating food that is processed, toxic and dangerous to your health—you'll find that your desire for sugar, oil and white flour will subside. You'll gain a new confidence in your ability to decide how you want to live, rather than being ruled by cravings. Each day will be a new adventure.

SUNDAYS: GET PREPPED
Do some meal preparation in advance: chop vegetables for salads/smoothies, make and freeze soups.

MONDAYS: GET ENERGIZED
Start the week with your favorite breakfast and make it special: set aside 15 minutes in the morning to sit down and savor the flavors.

TUESDAYS: GET INSPIRED
Find something you enjoy doing that doesn't involve food: take a walk, go window shopping, take a yoga class or just enjoy a little "me" time.

WEDNESDAYS: GET MOVING
Add some light exercise to your day: go for a walk, take the stairs instead of the elevator, or do some stretching.

THURSDAYS: GET CHALLENGED
Try something new, whether it's a recipe on the meal plan that calls for raw kale as a salad base, or a new route home from work.

FRIDAY: GET FOCUSED
The weekend is looming, with all of its social activities and unstructured free time. Plan out what you will be eating, and come up with strategies for dealing with social mealtimes.

SATURDAY: GET SOCIAL
Sticking to the 10 in 20 Detox Program doesn't mean you have to eat alone. Make brunch plans with your friends and opt for berries, oatmeal or a delicious salad.

DO I NEED SUPPLEMENTS?

When it comes to deciding which multivitamins and supplements to take, it is important to strive for micronutrient adequacy, while at the same time, avoiding harmful ingredients. Scientific studies indicate that certain nutrients – including vitamins A and E, beta carotene and folic acid – in isolated form, are harmful. Shockingly, almost all conventional supplements and multivitamins contain these ingredients – particularly vitamin A and folic acid – that may pose serious health risks and are associated with a potentially heightened risk of cancer and premature death.

It is critical to make sure that your multivitamin excludes these dangerous ingredients. It is also vitally important to make sure that your multivitamin includes the beneficial micronutrients that may be low, even on a healthful diet. These include vitamins D3, K2, and B12 and minerals zinc and iodine. In addition, the omega-3 fatty acids DHA and EPA are important for brain function, and anyone who doesn't regularly eat fish likely does not get enough. I advise against eating fish, especially because of the toxins they contain, and instead recommend an algae-derived omega-3 supplement for most people.

BENEFICIAL SUPPLEMENTS INCLUDE:

- **VITAMINS B12 AND K2** – which are produced by microorganisms and are difficult to obtain from plant food

- **ZINC** – which is difficult to absorb from plant sources

- **IODINE** – whose major dietary source is iodized salt

- **VEGAN VITAMIN D3** - which is the safest and most effective form of the "sunshine vitamin"

- **OMEGA 3 DHA AND EPA** – which are important for brain health

CHOOSING A SAFE MULTI

Most multivitamins contain ingredients that can be harmful to your health. Check the label to see if your supplement is doing more harm than good.

DO NOT TAKE VITAMINS THAT CONTAIN:

FOLIC ACID

Folic acid is a synthetic compound; folate is the natural form, with a different biological structure, found in natural foods and especially in green vegetables and beans. Avoid folic acid, as it's associated with increased risks of breast, prostate and colorectal cancers. Pregnancy use of folic acid is the biggest health mistake of modern history, as its use may increase the risk of childhood cancers, autism, and other serious health issues. Getting folate from natural produce, before and after conception, is "a must" for a healthy baby.

BETA CAROTENE

May interfere with absorption of other carotenoids. A study was halted due to significant increase of lung cancer in supplement users. Colorful fruits and vegetables supply hundreds of carotenoid compounds in complex forms, supplying maximum disease protection.

VITAMIN A

Studies suggest supplemental "A" causes loss of calcium in urine, weaker bones and increased risk of hip fracture. Excess can be dangerous, increasing risk of death; the body can make all it needs from carotenoids in plants.

VITAMIN E

Supplemental E is shown in various studies to increase risk of heart failure and all-cause mortality. Raw nuts and seeds supply complex Vitamin E forms in the healthiest fashion.

BE CAREFUL IF SUPPLEMENTING WITH THESE MINERALS:

SELENIUM

Helps regulate metabolism, but too much is linked to diabetes, elevated cholesterol, prostate cancer and cardiovascular disease.

COPPER

High intake is linked to increased risk of cancer, Alzheimer's, dementia and all-cause mortality.

IRON

Excess is linked to increased risk of cancer and heart disease.

IRON (FOR WOMEN)

Needs vary widely among women, and intake is best individualized according to ferritin levels. Pregnant women need sufficient iron for baby, but levels too high or too low can increase risk of low birth rate, oxidative stress and iron overload.

MAKE SURE YOUR MULTI CONTAINS THESE INGREDIENTS:

VITAMIN B12

Low levels are associated with increased risk of dementia, depression, fatigue, digestive issues and nerve damage. The RDI is inadequate for many. Vegans, flexitarians and the elderly may require 20 to 50 times more than the RDI.

ZINC

Essential for immune function, growth, skin health, wound healing, reproduction and insulin secretion. Phytates in plant foods bind zinc, making supplementation wise for vegans and near-vegans.

IODINE

Necessary for thyroid function and body metabolism. Both too much and too little can suppress thyroid function. A supplement (not iodinated salt) is safest, steady source.

VITAMIN D

Insufficient levels are linked with osteoporosis, cancer, diabetes, cardiovascular disease and depression. Vitamin D3 is most favorable form when supplementing.

VITAMIN K2

Essential for blood clotting and heart health; improves bone mineral density. K1 is abundant in green vegetables, but K2 is not found in plant foods, so supplementing with K2 is wise..

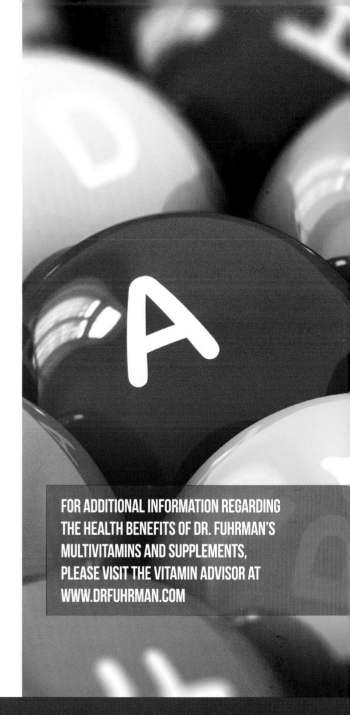

FOR ADDITIONAL INFORMATION REGARDING THE HEALTH BENEFITS OF DR. FUHRMAN'S MULTIVITAMINS AND SUPPLEMENTS, PLEASE VISIT THE VITAMIN ADVISOR AT WWW.DRFUHRMAN.COM

THE GROUND RULES

BEFORE YOU GET STARTED . . .

If you are hungry, you can eat more of the eat liberally (raw vegetables, cooked vegetables, beans and fruit) at mealtime, but stop eating before you feel full or stuffed. Try very hard not to eat even these eat liberally foods between mealtimes. Resist the urge to eat recreationally, or when you are not truly hungry.

Refer to Page 21 for Foods to Eat Liberally, Eat in Moderation or Avoid Entirely Food Chart

You can also eat larger portions or an extra portion of menu items that contain only unlimited foods.

The 10 in 20 Detox Program is based on eating large quantities of raw and cooked vegetables. These foods fill you up and leave little room for processed, refined foods which contain lots of calories but few nutrients. Eat a large salad. Some find it helpful to shoot for one pound of raw veggies each day. To give you a general idea, a pound of raw vegetables is a salad composed of: 5 cups of chopped romaine lettuce, 1 cup of shredded cabbage, 1 medium tomato, 1 small carrot and ¼ cup chopped raw onion. For cooked portions, 1 ½ cups of broccoli weighs about 8 ounces and 1 ½ cups of kale weighs 7 ounces.

Lunch and dinner recipes are interchangeable, so feel free to swap meals within these categories or repeat a meal more often than it is on the menu. When you have leftovers, they can be substituted for other meals. If you like a recipe, double it and freeze it in individual portions so you don't have to do as much cooking. Just don't have a meal that contains bread more than three times per week, and don't have a breakfast meal more than once a day. Recipes that include animal products (meat, eggs) should also be limited to three times per week.

Frozen vegetables or fruit can be substituted for fresh. Don't use canned vegetables or fruit. Canned products lose nutrients during processing and often contain added sugar or salt.

As you change your diet and discontinue unhealthy, addictive foods, your body may go through a detox or

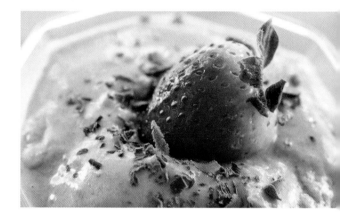

withdrawal phase where you feel weak or uncomfortable, or experience cravings for certain foods. This means that your body is healing and the removal of toxins is underway. These symptoms will start to resolve gradually as you flood your body with high-nutrient, whole plant foods.

Your stomach doesn't have teeth, so chew your food well. It takes the digestive tract time to adjust to a high-fiber diet that contains lots of raw vegetables and beans. Chewing well helps to ease the digestive process, and also ensures that more nutrients are available for absorption.

FOODS TO EAT LIBERALLY, EAT IN MODERATION OR AVOID ENTIRELY

Whether you want to lose weight or just eat more healthfully, an easy way to make the right dietary choices is to sort foods into three categories: those you may eat liberally, those you should eat in moderation, or those you should avoid entirely. Note that the term "eat liberally" is more accurate than the term "unlimited." Unlimited could imply overeating, or recreational or emotional eating, or eating when not hungry. Also, consuming too much of a very healthy food, such as fruit, can lead to insufficient vegetables in your diet.

FOLLOW THESE GUIDELINES:

EAT LIBERALLY
You can eat as much as you want of these foods: (within reason):
- **Raw vegetables** *(Goal: about ½ to 1 pound daily)*
- **Cooked green and non-green nutrient–dense vegetables** *(Goal: about ½ to 1 pound daily)*
Non-green nutrient dense veggies are: tomatoes, cauliflower, eggplant, mushrooms, peppers, onions and carrots
- **Beans, legumes, tofu, lentils, tempeh and edamame** *(Goal: ½-1 cup daily)*

LIMITED (EAT IN MODERATION)
Include these foods in your diet, but limit the amount you are eating:
- **Fresh or frozen fruit** *(Maximum: 5 servings daily, one should be berries)*
- **Cooked starchy vegetables or whole grains**
(Maximum: 2 servings daily; 1 serving = 1 cup or 1 slice)
  - Butternut and other winter squashes
  - Sweet potatoes *(avoid white potatoes)*, corn or wild rice
  - Quinoa or other intact whole grains
  - 100% whole grain bread
- **Raw nuts and seeds.** Half should be walnuts or chia, hemp, flax or sesame seeds *(Maximum: women 2 ounces or men 3 ounces)*
- **Avocado** *(Maximum ½ per day)*
- **Dried Fruit** *(Maximum 2 tablespoons per day)*
- **Animal Products: fat-free dairy, clean wild fish and certified organic poultry** *(Maximum of 6 ounces per week, limit each serving size to 2 ounces and use as a minor component/flavoring agent)*

Note: If you are not trying to lose weight, amounts of cooked starchy vegetables, intact whole grains, nuts, seeds and avocado may be moderately increased depending on your caloric needs.

OFF-LIMITS (AVOID ENTIRELY)
- **Products made with sugar or white flour**
- **Soda and soft drinks** including those made with artificial sweeteners
- **Fruit Juice**
- **Barbequed, processed and cured meats and all red meat**
- **Full-fat and reduced-fat dairy** *(cheese, ice cream, butter, milk)*
- **Eggs**
- **All vegetable oils, including olive oil and coconut oil**

Note: If you are not trying to lose weight, a small amount of olive oil, a teaspoon a day or less may be used.

STOCK YOUR PANTRY

Before you begin the meal plan, clean out your refrigerator and cabinets of all trigger foods or designate a space for your healthy foods. Stock your pantry with these staple items. They will be needed for the recipes and meals you will be preparing for the next 20 days. Four additional shopping lists are also included with the menus. These are compiled for five-day time periods and include perishable items and other foods specific to each set of menus.

NUTS AND SEEDS

All nuts and seeds should be raw and unsalted
Walnuts
Almonds
Cashews
Ground flax seeds
Whole chia seeds
Pumpkin seeds
Sunflower seeds
Unhulled sesame seeds
Raw almond butter
Raw cashew butter

DRIED HERBS AND SPICES

No-salt seasoning blend such as Mrs. Dash
Onion powder
Garlic powder
Chili powder
Cumin
Curry powder
Dried oregano
Dried basil
Dried thyme
Dried rosemary
Allspice

Sweet paprika
Black pepper
Red pepper flakes
Ground red cayenne pepper
Cinnamon
Vanilla extract

WHOLE GRAINS, DRIED FRUIT, VINEGARS AND OTHER ITEMS

Old fashioned rolled oats and steel cut oats
Quinoa and/or other intact whole grain such as farro
Bulgur (quinoa may be substituted)
Wild rice
100% whole grain flour tortillas such as Ezekiel or Alvarado Street brands (store in freezer)
100% whole grain pitas such as Ezekiel or Alvarado Street brands (store in freezer)
Dates
Raisins
Unsweetened dried coconut
Natural, non-alkalized cocoa powder
Nutritional yeast
Bragg's Liquid Aminos or low-sodium soy sauce
Balsamic vinegar
Rice vinegar
Fig-flavored vinegar such as Dr. Fuhrman's Black Fig Vinegar
Dijon Mustard

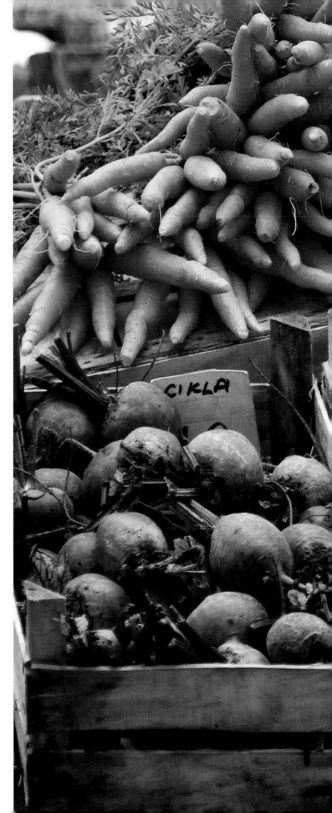

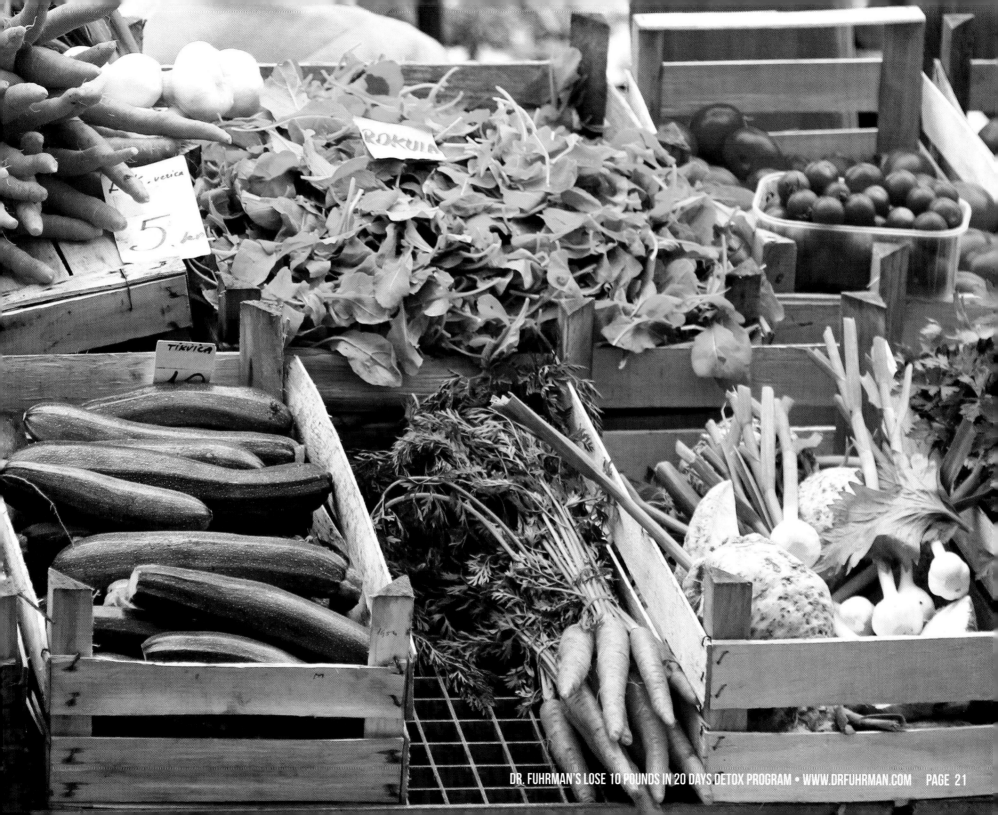

DAYS 1-5
SHOPPING LIST

This shopping list assumes that all recipes in the meal plan will be made. Menus frequently include fruit for dessert and will mention a specific fruit as an example. That fruit is used for the shopping list.

Make sure you also have all the items listed in the Stock Your Pantry list.

FRESH PRODUCE

VEGETABLES

- [ ] 3 heads romaine lettuce
- [ ] 1 head Boston lettuce (optional, could use some of the romaine)
- [ ] 8 cups mixed greens (about 8 ounces)
- [ ] 2 bunches kale
- [ ] 10 ounces spinach (could also buy frozen)
- [ ] Your choice of a green vegetable to equal 2 cups cooked (could also buy frozen)
- [ ] 2-3 crowns broccoli (about 2 cups florets) (could also buy frozen)
- [ ] 1 small red cabbage
- [ ] 6 medium tomatoes
- [ ] Pint cherry tomatoes
- [ ] 3 avocados
- [ ] 2 medium zucchini
- [ ] 1 medium cucumber
- [ ] 2 green bell peppers

- [ ] 1 Portobello mushroom
- [ ] 7 ounces white or cremini mushrooms
- [ ] 1 sweet or Spanish onion
- [ ] 4 yellow onions
- [ ] 2 red onions
- [ ] 1 head garlic
- [ ] Fresh basil
- [ ] Fresh cilantro

FRUIT

- [ ] 2 pints (about 4 cups) blueberries (could also buy 20 ounces of frozen blueberries)
- [ ] 1 pound strawberries (could also buy frozen)
- [ ] 3 (4 for men) apples
- [ ] 2 (3 for men) navel oranges
- [ ] 2 bananas
- [ ] Small bunch grapes
- [ ] 2 lemons
- [ ] 1 lime

REFRIGERATED

- [ ] 3 cups unsweetened soy, hemp or almond milk. You can use all unflavored or if desired, use vanilla unsweetened for breakfast and smoothies and unflavored, unsweetened for other recipes. (1 cup must be unflavored; 2 cups can be either unflavored or vanilla)
- [ ] Small package non-dairy mozzarella-type cheese, optional

FROZEN

This list does not include foods that have a frozen option on the Fresh Produce list.

- [ ] 12 ounces (need 2 ⅓ cups) frozen corn
- [ ] 16 ounces (need 3 cups) frozen broccoli
- [ ] 10 ounces (need 1 cup) frozen artichoke hearts (If you can't find artichokes, substitute Brussels sprouts)
- [ ] 10 ounces (need 1 ½ cups) frozen cherries

SHELF STABLE

BEANS

It is assumed that canned low sodium or no-salt-added beans will be used. If you opt to start with dry beans, 1 cup of dry beans will yield about 3 cups of cooked beans

- [ ] 3 (15 ounce) cans kidney beans
- [ ] 1 (15 ounce) can black beans
- [ ] 2 (15 ounce) cans chick peas
- [ ] Add extra 2 (15 ounce) cans any variety for men

OTHER

Choose tomato products packaged in cartons or glass. These materials do not contain BPA.

- [ ] 1 (15 ounce) can low sodium or no-salt-added vegetable broth
- [ ] 1 (26 ounce carton) low-sodium diced tomatoes
- [ ] Low-sodium pasta sauce (need ½ cup)
- [ ] Low-sodium salsa (need ½ cup)

DAY 1

A magic ratio of carbohydrate, fat and protein that will lead you to your ideal weight and superior health does not exist. Good health and weight control are the result of major changes in the nutritional quality of the foods you eat. It is the nutritional quality and healthfulness of those carbs, fat and protein that will determine your health. The ratio (within reason, of course) does not matter.

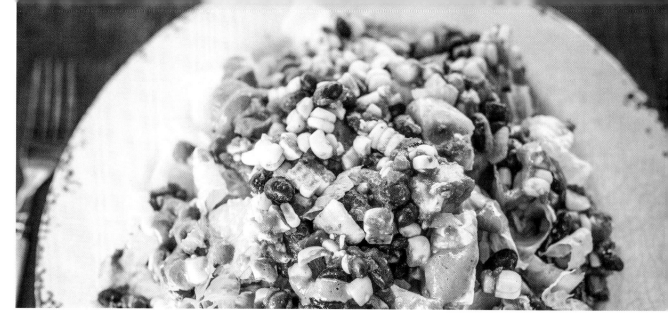

BREAKFAST
SOAKED OATS AND BLUEBERRIES
1 SERVING

½ cup uncooked old fashioned oats

½ cup unsweetened, unflavored or vanilla soy, hemp or almond milk

½ cup blueberries

1 small apple, chopped

½ tablespoon ground flax seeds

Combine oats and non-dairy milk. Soak for at least 30 minutes or overnight. Mix in remaining ingredients.

Men: Add ¼ cup chopped raw nuts/seeds

LUNCH
MEXICAN SALAD
1 SERVING

1 head romaine lettuce, chopped

½ cup cooked black beans

⅓ cup frozen, thawed corn kernels

¼ cup low sodium salsa

½ avocado, peeled and chopped

Toss lettuce with beans, corn and salsa. Top your salad with the chopped avocado. (Wrap up the other avocado half, refrigerate and save for tomorrow)

If you use canned beans, choose low sodium or no-salt-added varieties. Save the leftover beans — you can use them later in the week.

Orange or other fruit for dessert

DINNER
EASY VEGETABLE PIZZA
1 SERVING

1 large (100% whole grain) tortilla or pita

½ cup low sodium pasta sauce

¼ cup chopped mushrooms

¼ cup chopped red onion

1 cup frozen broccoli, thawed and chopped

1 tablespoon shredded non-dairy mozzarella-type cheese, optional

Preheat oven to 200 degrees F. Place tortilla on a baking sheet and warm for 10 minutes. Remove from oven and top with remaining ingredients. Bake for 30 minutes.

If you are following a gluten-free diet, substitute a dinner item from another night.

Your choice of a cooked green vegetable or a mixed green salad with tomatoes, onions, other veggies and Easy Balsamic Almond Dressing

Steam or water sauté fresh vegetables. If desired, sauté with fresh chopped garlic or onion. Season with lemon, balsamic vinegar and/or your choice of herbs, spices or a no-salt seasoning blend. For some heat, add red pepper flakes, cayenne pepper, or black pepper.

> **Tip:** Frozen vegetables are a convenient option. They are rich in micronutrients because they are picked ripe and flash-frozen soon after picking. It is fine to substitute frozen vegetables for fresh.

EASY BALSAMIC ALMOND DRESSING
1 SERVING

2 tablespoons water

1 tablespoon plus 1 teaspoon balsamic vinegar

1 tablespoon raw almond butter

¼ teaspoon onion powder

¼ teaspoon garlic powder

⅛ teaspoon dried oregano

⅛ teaspoon dried basil

Whisk water, vinegar and almond butter together until mixture is smooth and almond butter is evenly dispersed. Mix in remaining ingredients.

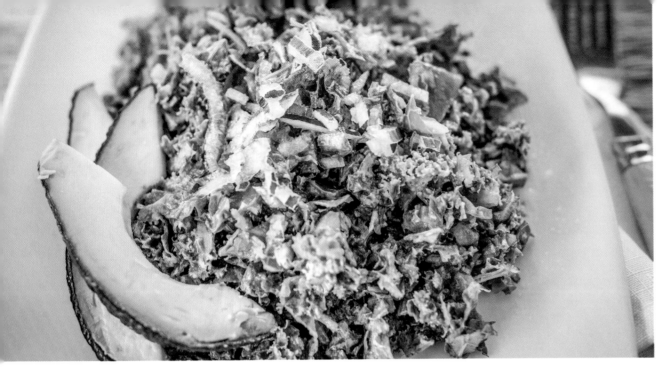

DAY 2

Vegetables, especially green leafy vegetables, win the nutrient density prize. The concentration of vitamins, minerals, phytochemicals and antioxidants per calorie in vegetables is the highest, by far, of any food.

BREAKFAST
BERRY BOWL
1 SERVING

1 ½ cups fresh (or thawed frozen) blueberries, strawberries, blackberries and/or raspberries

1 banana, sliced

¼ cup unsweetened, unflavored or vanilla soy, hemp or almond milk

2 tablespoons chopped walnuts

1 tablespoon ground flax or chia seeds

Top berries and sliced banana with non-dairy milk and sprinkle with walnuts and the flax or chia seeds.

Men: Increase chopped walnuts to ¼ cup

LUNCH
KALE AVOCADO SALAD
1 SERVING

1 small bunch kale, shredded (about 5 cups)

½ avocado, chopped

½ lemon, juiced

1 small tomato, diced

2 tablespoons red onion, diced

¼ teaspoon Bragg Liquid Aminos or low sodium soy sauce

Pinch cayenne pepper

Toss ingredients together in a bowl, squeezing as you mix to wilt the kale and cream the avocado.

Men: Add a cup of cooked quinoa or farro to the salad or have the whole avocado

Grapes or other fruit for dessert

DINNER
ZUCCHINI SPAGHETTI WITH FRESH TOMATO SAUCE
1 SERVING

2 zucchini

½ sweet onion, chopped

2 garlic cloves, chopped

1 cup sliced mushrooms

2 tomatoes, chopped

Fresh basil, if desired

Using a vegetable peeler or a vegetable spiralizer, cut zucchini into thin pieces to resemble spaghetti or simply cut into thin slices. Place zucchini in a colander to drain excess moisture. Meanwhile, heat 2-3 tablespoons of water in a pan and sauté the onion for a minute, then add the garlic and mushrooms and cook until tender. Add tomatoes and if you like, some fresh basil and cook for another 5 minutes. Top the zucchini linguini with the tomato sauce.

If you prefer cooked zucchini, add it to the tomato sauce during the last 2-3 minutes of cooking.

Men: Add ½ -1 cup cooked or low-sodium canned beans

CHOCOLATE CHERRY ICE CREAM
2 SERVINGS

½ cup unsweetened unflavored or vanilla soy, hemp or almond milk

1 tablespoon natural cocoa powder

4 regular dates, pitted

1 ½ cups frozen dark sweet cherries

Blend ingredients in a high-powered blender.

Freeze leftover ice cream and enjoy it over the next few days – whenever you need a dessert treat.

DAY 3

Don't give in to food addictions. After the first week, junk food withdrawal will subside and you will learn to prefer the fresh, natural flavors of whole foods.

BREAKFAST

ORANGE AND KALE SMOOTHIE
1 SERVING

1½ cups kale, tough stems and ribs removed

1 apple, cored and sliced

1 navel orange, peeled

½ lemon, juiced

1 tablespoon ground flax seeds

2-3 ice cubes

Blend ingredients in a high-powered blender.

Men: Add an extra ¼ cup raw nuts and/or seeds

LUNCH

HUMMUS WRAP
1 SERVING

1 large (100% whole grain) tortilla

3 tablespoons hummus (see note)

½ cup chopped romaine, ½ cup sliced tomatoes and 2 slices red onion

Splash balsamic vinegar

Spread hummus on the wrap, top with chopped romaine, diced tomatoes, sliced red onion and a splash of balsamic vinegar

Gluten-free option: substitute a few large Swiss chard or collard leaves for the tortilla

Note: To make oil-free, no-salt-added hummus, blend 1½ cups cooked chickpeas, 2 tablespoons lemon juice, 2 tablespoons unhulled sesame seeds, 1 garlic clove and ½ teaspoon cumin in a food processor or high-powered blender. Add 1–2 tablespoons water if need to adjust consistency.

Thawed frozen cherries or other fruit for dessert

DINNER

SALAD WITH MIXED BABY GREENS, TOMATOES, ONIONS, SHREDDED RED CABBAGE AND EASY BALSAMIC ALMOND DRESSING

(recipe from Day 1 dinner)

Tip: If you are pressed for time and opt for a bottled dressing, use a no-oil dressing that contains no more than 75 mg of sodium per tablespoon. Add 1 to 2 tablespoons of raw nuts or seeds to enhance the absorption of nutrients from the salad.

TAILGATE CHILI
5 SERVINGS

½ cup uncooked bulgur or quinoa

1 cup water

3 cups chopped onions

3 cloves garlic, minced

2 green bell peppers, chopped

26 ounces low sodium diced tomatoes (see note)

3 (15 ounce) cans red kidney beans, no salt added or low sodium, rinsed and drained

2 cups fresh or frozen corn kernels

2 tablespoons chili powder

2 teaspoons ground cumin

Combine bulgur or quinoa and water in a saucepan. Bring to a boil, reduce heat and simmer for 12 to 15 minutes or until tender.

Meanwhile, heat ⅛ cup water in a large saucepan and water sauté onions and garlic until almost soft, about 5 minutes. Stir in green peppers and sauté an additional 3 minutes, adding more water as needed. Stir in diced tomatoes, beans, corn, chili powder and cumin. Bring to a boil, reduce heat, cover and simmer for 20 minutes. Add bulgur or quinoa and simmer for an additional 5 minutes.

Note: Choose tomato products packaged in cartons or glass. These materials do not contain BPA.

Men: Have an extra serving of chili

Portion leftover chili into individual containers. If you like, you can have another serving tomorrow for lunch. Use the remaining servings for alternate lunches or dinners over the next 3 to 4 days if you are short on time, or freeze for later use.

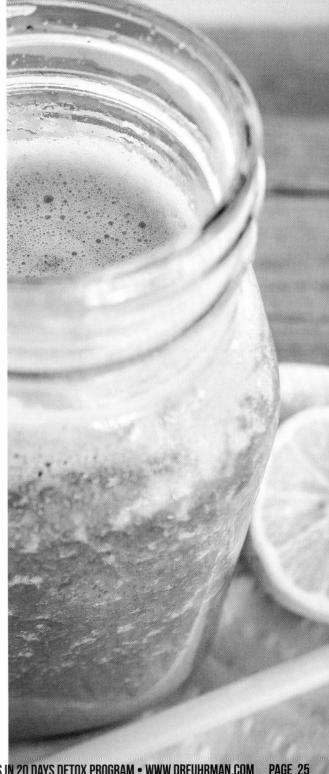

DAY 4

Avoid foods that are completely empty of nutrients or toxic to the body, such as sugar and other refined sweeteners, white flour, processed foods and fast foods.

BREAKFAST

CHIA SEED BREAKFAST PUDDING
1 SERVING

½ cup unsweetened, unflavored or vanilla soy, hemp or almond milk

2 tablespoons whole chia seeds

2 tablespoons uncooked old fashioned or steel cut oats

½ banana, sliced *(peel and freeze the other half — you will use it to make a healthy ice cream)*

½ cup fresh blueberries or frozen, thawed

In a bowl, mix together non-dairy milk, chia seeds and oats. Let mixture sit for 10 minutes or for an on-the-run breakfast, make the night before and refrigerate. Stir in banana and blueberries.

Note: If using steel cut oats, make the night before.

Men: Add an Orange and Kale Smoothie (See Day 3)

LUNCH

> **Tip:** Instead of low-nutrient, refined oils, use real foods such as walnuts, sesame seeds, other nuts, seeds and avocado as the fat sources in your salad dressings.

PORTOBELLO SALAD WITH WALNUT VINAIGRETTE (OR LEFTOVER CHILI FROM LAST NIGHT)
SALAD: 1 SERVING   DRESSING: 4 SERVINGS

1 Portobello mushroom

5 cups mixed greens

¼ cup sliced red onion

½ cucumber, sliced

6 cherry tomatoes

For the Walnut Vinaigrette:

¼ cup balsamic vinegar

½ cup water

¼ cup walnuts

¼ cup raisins

1 teaspoon Dijon mustard

1 clove garlic

¼ teaspoon dried thyme

Slice the Portobello mushroom and sauté in water or vegetable broth (or grill it). Toss together mixed greens, onion, cucumber and tomatoes. Top with the sliced mushroom.

For the dressing, combine all ingredients in a high-powered blender. Drizzle desired amount of dressing over salad.

Men: Add 1 cup beans and ¼ cup raw nuts/seeds

Store the remaining dressing in the fridge; you will use it on Day 6.

Melon or other fruit for dessert

DINNER

CHICKPEA CURRY IN A HURRY
2 SERVINGS

1½ cups cooked chickpeas or 1 (15 ounce) can low sodium chickpeas, drained

½ cup low-sodium vegetable broth

1 ½ cups diced tomatoes

1 teaspoon garlic powder

2 teaspoons curry powder

⅓ cup unsweetened dried coconut

1 10-ounce box or bag frozen chopped spinach

Combine all ingredients except spinach in a large saucepan. Cook for 5 minutes, then add spinach. Cover and continue cooking until spinach is thawed and curry is warm, about 5 more minutes.

Enjoy one serving now and save one for lunch tomorrow or another time when you are too busy to cook.

Serve with 1 cup cooked quinoa, farro or other intact whole grain

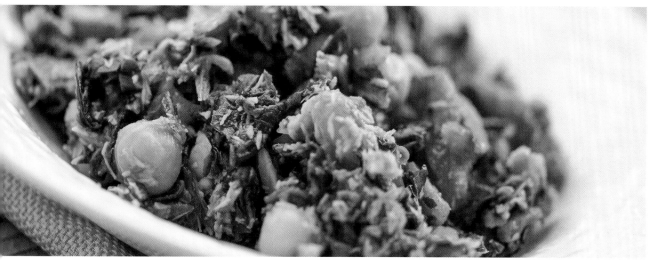

DAY 5

Never eat to the point that you feel full.
Stop eating before you feel uncomfortable.
Three-quarters of the way through a meal,
stand up and walk around to make sure you are
not overeating.

BREAKFAST

APPLE PIE OATMEAL
1 SERVING

¼ cup old fashioned or steel cut oats

½ cup water

1 apple, peeled, cored, and diced

dash cinnamon

1-2 tablespoons raisins or currants

2 tablespoons chopped walnuts

Combine oats and water in a small pot, bring to a boil, then
reduce heat and simmer for 5 minutes. Stir in remaining ingredients.

Note: If using steel cut oats, double the amount of water and
simmer for 20 minutes or until tender.

Men: Add a banana

LUNCH

BLACK BEAN LETTUCE BUNDLES
1 SERVING

1 cup cooked or canned low-sodium black beans, drained

⅓ ripe avocado, peeled, pitted and mashed

2 tablespoons chopped fresh cilantro

¼ cup mild, no-salt-added or low-sodium salsa

1 tablespoon fresh lime juice

1 clove garlic, minced

½ teaspoon ground cumin

4-5 large Boston lettuce or romaine leaves

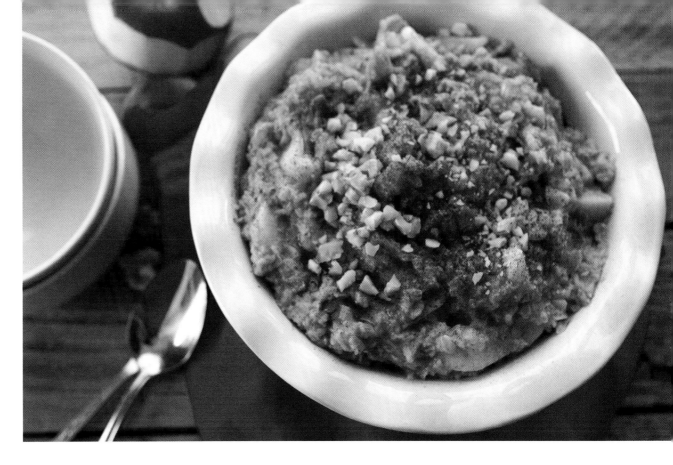

In a bowl, mash the beans and avocado together with a fork until
well blended and only slightly chunky. Add all the remaining
ingredients except the lettuce and mix.

Place some of the mixture in the center of each lettuce leaf and
roll up like a burrito.

Fresh or thawed frozen berries for dessert

DINNER

CREAMY KALE AND MUSHROOM CASSEROLE
4 SERVINGS

½ cup raw cashews or ¼ cup raw cashew butter

1 cup unsweetened, unflavored soy, hemp or almond milk

2 cups small fresh or frozen broccoli florets

1 cup chopped mushrooms

1 cup frozen artichoke hearts, thawed and chopped (see note)

2 cups chopped kale, tough stems removed

1 teaspoon no-salt seasoning blend such as Mrs. Dash

1 teaspoon onion powder

1 teaspoon garlic powder

¼ teaspoon red pepper flakes

Preheat oven to 350 degrees.

Blend the cashews and non-dairy milk until creamy. Add to a 9x13
inch oven-proof baking dish along with broccoli, mushrooms,
artichokes, kale, and seasonings. Bake for 40 minutes.

Note: Frozen Brussels sprouts may be substituted for the
artichoke hearts

Men: Have 2 servings of Kale and Mushroom Casserole

*Refrigerate leftover casserole or freeze in individual portions and
use for a quick and easy alternate lunch or dinner.*

DAYS 6-10
SHOPPING LIST

This shopping list assumes that all recipes in the meal plan will be made. Menus frequently include fruit for dessert and will mention a specific fruit as an example. That fruit is used for the shopping list.

Check your refrigerator, freezer and pantry before shopping. You may have items leftover from Days 1-5 that you can use. Make sure you also have all the items listed in the Stock Your Pantry list.

FRESH PRODUCE

VEGETABLES

- [ ] 3 heads romaine lettuce
- [ ] 10 cups mixed greens (about 10 ounces)
- [ ] 2 bunches kale
- [ ] 5 ounces spinach (7 ounces for men)
- [ ] Your choice of a green or other high nutrient vegetable such as cauliflower, mushrooms or butternut squash to equal 2 cups cooked (could also buy frozen)
- [ ] 1-2 broccoli crowns
- [ ] 1 cup cauliflower florets
- [ ] 1 small red cabbage
- [ ] 6 medium tomatoes
- [ ] 3 avocados
- [ ] 1 medium zucchini
- [ ] 3 red peppers
- [ ] 2 medium cucumbers
- [ ] ½ cup snow peas
- [ ] 2 Portobello mushrooms
- [ ] 7 ounces white or cremini mushrooms

- [ ] Shiitake mushrooms (need 1 cup sliced)
- [ ] 1 sweet potato
- [ ] 6 carrots
- [ ] 11 stalks celery
- [ ] 1 red onion
- [ ] 4 yellow onions
- [ ] 2 scallions (green onions)
- [ ] 6 cloves garlic (any leftover from Days 1-5?)
- [ ] 1 small piece fresh ginger

FRUIT

- [ ] 2 pints (about 4 cups) blueberries (or 20 ounces of frozen blueberries)
- [ ] 5 bananas
- [ ] 2 navel oranges
- [ ] 1 pear or Granny Smith apple
- [ ] 2 (3 for men) ripe mangos (or 16-24 ounces frozen mango)
- [ ] Small bunch grapes
- [ ] 1 lime
- [ ] Add extra 3 cups of fruit for men

REFRIGERATED

- [ ] 1 ¼ cups unsweetened, unflavored or vanilla soy, hemp or almond milk
- [ ] ⅓ cup pomegranate juice or ½ cup pomegranate kernels
- [ ] 7 ounces extra firm tofu
- [ ] Non-dairy yogurt, optional
- [ ] 4 ounces ground organic turkey, optional (for vegan Black Bean Burgers, purchase an additional 15-ounce can of black beans)
- [ ] 2 ounces chicken breast, optional
- [ ] 1 egg, optional

FROZEN

This list does not include foods that have a frozen option on the Fresh Produce list.

- [ ] 1 cup frozen corn (any leftover from days 1-5?)
- [ ] 1 cup frozen cherries (any leftover from days 1-5?)

SHELF STABLE

BEANS

It is assumed that canned low sodium or no-salt-added beans will be used. If you opt to start with dry beans, 1 cup of dry beans will yield about 3 cups of cooked beans.

- [ ] 3 (15 ounce) cans black beans
- [ ] ½ cup yellow split peas
- [ ] ½ cup shelled edamame or other cooked/canned bean
- [ ] Add extra 2 (15 ounce) cans any variety for men

OTHER

Choose tomato products packaged in cartons or glass. These materials do not contain BPA.

- [ ] Low sodium or no-salt-added vegetable juice or carrot juice (need 2 cups)
- [ ] Low sodium tomato sauce (need 1 ½ cups)
- [ ] Low sodium pasta sauce (need ¼ cup)
- [ ] Low sodium salsa (need 1 cup)
- [ ] ¼-½ cup coconut water (optional instead of non-dairy milk in Day 7 smoothie)

DAY 6

Always keep an assortment of healthful foods available. When you leave home for work or play, pack food to take with you so that you are not stranded with unhealthy choices.

BREAKFAST

BLENDED MANGO SALAD
1 SERVING

1 ripe mango, peeled and chopped or 1 ½ cups frozen mango chunks

2 cups spinach

1 cup chopped romaine lettuce

¼ cup unsweetened, unflavored or vanilla non-dairy milk or coconut water

½ tablespoon ground flax seeds

Blend ingredients in a high-powered blender or food processor.

Men: Add 1 cup cooked steel cut or old fashioned oats with non-dairy milk and fresh or thawed frozen fruit.

LUNCH

MIXED GREENS SALAD WITH PEARS, APPLES AND WALNUT VINAIGRETTE (or leftover Chickpea Curry or Creamy Kale and Mushroom Casserole)
SALAD: 1 SERVING   DRESSING: 4 SERVINGS

2 cups mixed salad greens

2 cups chopped romaine lettuce

1 small ripe pear or Granny Smith apple, cubed

¼ cup thinly sliced red onion

2 tablespoons raw pumpkin seeds, lightly toasted

For the Walnut Vinaigrette: (any left over from Day 4?)

¼ cup balsamic vinegar

½ cup water

¼ cup walnuts

½ cup raisins

1 teaspoon Dijon mustard

1 small clove garlic

Toss salad ingredients together. To make dressing, combine dressing ingredients in a high-powered blender.

DINNER

Tip: If you are pressed for time, you can use store-bought frozen veggie burgers. Select a product that does not contain isolated soy protein and is labeled low sodium or light in sodium.

TURKEY BURGERS WITH BLACK BEANS AND MUSHROOMS
4 SERVINGS

(Vegan option: Black Bean and Mushroom Burgers)

1 cup chopped mushrooms

¼ cup old fashioned rolled oats

2 tablespoons raw pumpkin seeds

1 carrot, grated

1 cup cooked or canned low sodium black beans, drained

¼ teaspoon cumin

¼ teaspoon chili powder

¼ teaspoon onion powder

⅛ teaspoon black pepper

4 ounces ground organic turkey (For vegan burgers, omit turkey and use an additional cup of beans)

Preheat oven to 300 degrees F.

Heat 1-2 tablespoons water in a small pan and sauté mushrooms until tender and moisture has evaporated, about 5 minutes. Set aside.

Grind oats and pumpkin seeds in a food processor. Add grated carrots, ¾ cup of the beans (1 ¾ cups for vegan burgers) and all of the spices and process until blended.

Spoon mixture into a mixing bowl and stir in sautéed mushrooms, remaining ¼ cup whole beans and ground turkey. Form into 4 medium sized patties. Place on a baking sheet lined with parchment paper or lightly wiped with olive oil. Bake for 40 minutes, turning once after 20 minutes.

Serve on a bed of mixed greens with sliced red onion and tomato or on a small 100% whole grain roll or pita with onion, tomato and lettuce.

Men: Have an extra burger without the roll and add ½ avocado, sliced

Refrigerate or freeze leftover patties for another meal or enjoy your burgers with a friend. Save leftover beans; you will use them another night.

BANANA WALNUT ICE CREAM
2 SERVINGS

Do-ahead: peel two ripe bananas, wrap in plastic wrap and freeze

2 ripe bananas, frozen

⅓ cup unsweetened, unflavored or vanilla non-dairy milk

2 tablespoons walnuts

Place bananas, non-dairy milk and 2 tablespoons walnuts in a high-powered blender and blend until smooth and creamy.

Eat one serving now and freeze the other serving. Enjoy it over the next few days-whenever you need a dessert treat.

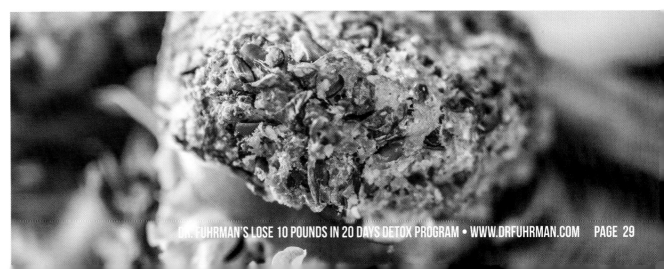

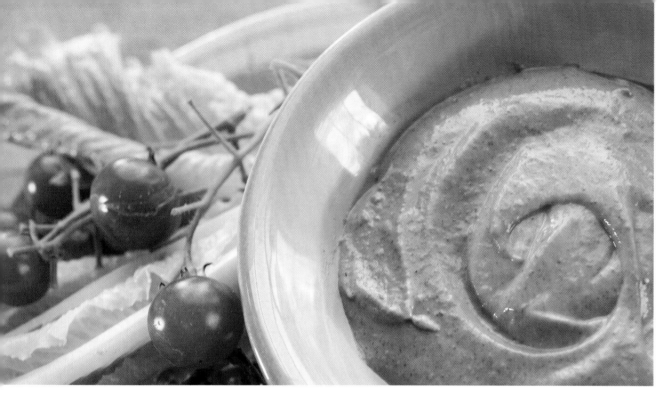

DAY 7

Eating a large amount of greens and other colorful vegetables is the secret weapon to achieving good health and your ideal body weight.

BREAKFAST

BANANA CASHEW LETTUCE WRAPS
1 SERVING

2 tablespoons raw cashew butter
6 Boston lettuce or romaine lettuce leaves
1 banana, thinly sliced

Spread about 1 teaspoon cashew butter on each lettuce leaf. Lay a few banana slices on the butter and roll up like a burrito.

Men: Add the Blended Mango Salad (see Day 6 Breakfast).

LUNCH

BIG GREEN SALAD WITH RUSSIAN DRESSING

Include tomatoes, red onions, shredded red cabbage, other veggies and ½ cup shelled edamame or other cooked beans

RUSSIAN DRESSING
2 SERVINGS

4 tablespoons low sodium pasta sauce
3 tablespoons raw almond butter or ⅓ cup raw almonds
2 tablespoons balsamic vinegar or Dr. Fuhrman's Black Fig Vinegar

Blend together with a fork or whisk if using almond butter. If using raw almonds, blend in a high-powered blender.

Save leftover Russian Dressing for your Tomato Almond Pita Pocket on Day 9

Orange or other fruit for dessert

DINNER

> **Tip:** Get in the habit of making a pot of soup once or twice a week. It is easy to incorporate a variety of green leafy vegetables, mushrooms, onions, beans and other healthy ingredients all in one pot. When vegetables are simmered in soup, all the nutrients are retained in the liquid and the gentle heat prevents nutrient loss. Soups also make great leftovers.

CHEESY KALE SOUP
4 SERVINGS

½ cup dry yellow split peas
1 onion, chopped
1 cup mushrooms, sliced
2 cups carrot juice or low sodium vegetable broth
1½ cups low sodium tomato sauce
5 cups chopped kale
⅓ cup raw cashew butter or ⅔ cup raw cashews
2 tablespoons nutritional yeast

Bring 2 cups of water to a boil, add the split peas and simmer until tender, about 35-40 minutes. Add onion, mushrooms, carrot juice or broth and tomato sauce. Bring to a boil, reduce heat, then add kale. Cover and simmer until tender, about 15 minutes, adding a little water if you want to adjust the consistency. Stir in cashew butter and nutritional yeast. If using whole cashews, place in a blender and blend with ½ cup of the soup liquid, then return to the pot.

Men: Have 2 servings of soup

Refrigerate leftover soup or freeze in individual portions and use for a quick and easy alternate lunch or dinner.

Grapes or other fruit for dessert

DAY 8

The villain is not fat in general, but rather oils, saturated fats, trans fats and the fats consumed in processed foods. The good fats from nuts, seeds and avocados are rich in antioxidants and phytochemicals and offer unique health benefits.

BREAKFAST

TOFU SCRAMBLE (WITH OPTIONAL EGG)
1 SERVING

2 scallions, diced
¼ cup finely chopped red bell pepper
1 small tomato, chopped
1 clove garlic, minced or pressed
7 ounces extra firm tofu, drained and crumbled (reduce to 3½ ounces if using an egg)
1 egg, beaten, optional
½ teaspoon no-salt seasoning blend such as Mrs. Dash
1 tablespoon nutritional yeast
3 cups coarsely chopped spinach

Sauté scallions, red pepper, tomato, and garlic in ¼ cup water for 5 minutes. Add tofu, egg if desired, no-salt seasoning blend, nutritional yeast and spinach and cook for another 2 minutes.

May be served with low sodium ketchup or salsa. For some heat, add some hot pepper flakes.

Men: Have 2 cups fresh or thawed frozen fruit topped with flax, hemp or chia seeds

> **Tip:** Dry beans are more economical than canned beans. One cup of dry beans will yield 3 cups of cooked beans.

LUNCH

MICRO CHOPPED SALAD (or leftover soup)
1 SERVING

1 carrot, peeled
2 stalks celery
½ small onion
1 head romaine
1 tomato
½ avocado, peeled and cubed

Optional ingredients: cilantro, fresh lime juice, basil, roasted garlic

Cut vegetables into large chunks. Add carrots, celery and onion to a food processor with an S blade. Process until chopped in small pieces, then add the lettuce, process until chopped, then add the tomato and continue to process until everything is chopped in very small pieces. If you don't have a food processor, no problem—just chop it by hand.

Cut the avocado into cubes and mix with the chopped ingredients. Add optional ingredients as desired.

Men: Mix 1 cup cooked or low sodium canned beans and 2 tablespoons chopped walnuts into chopped salad.

Fresh or thawed frozen berries for dessert

DINNER

RAW VEGGIES WITH ORANGE PEANUT DIP

ORANGE PEANUT DIP
2 SERVINGS

1 orange, peeled and seeded
2 tablespoons rice vinegar
⅛ cup natural peanut butter, no salt added
1 tablespoon unhulled sesame seeds
½ teaspoon Bragg Liquid Aminos or low sodium soy sauce
1 teaspoon chopped fresh ginger

Blend all ingredients in a high-powered blender until smooth.

Save leftover dip for dinner on Day 10.

SWEET POTATOES TOPPED WITH BLACK BEANS AND KALE
1 SERVING

1 large sweet potato
¼ cup chopped onion
1 clove garlic, chopped
2 cups chopped kale
1 cup cooked or canned low sodium black beans, drained
1 cup diced tomatoes
½ teaspoon chili powder
¼ teaspoon cumin
2 tablespoons non-dairy yogurt, optional

Pierce sweet potato in several spots with a fork. Microwave on high until soft, 8-10 minutes. It can also be baked in a 350 degree F oven for 45 minutes or until soft.

Meanwhile, heat 2 tablespoons water in a large pan and water sauté onion and garlic for a minute, then add kale and stir until wilted. Cover pan and cook until kale is tender, adding water as needed, about 10 minutes. Add black beans, tomatoes, chili powder and cumin, bring to a simmer and cook for 5 minutes.

Cut potato lengthwise, remove skin and partially mash, then top with bean mixture. Sprinkle with cilantro and if desired, top with non-diary yogurt.

Save leftover beans; you will use them another night.

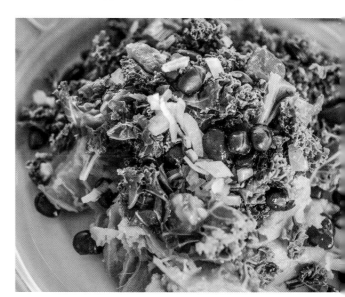

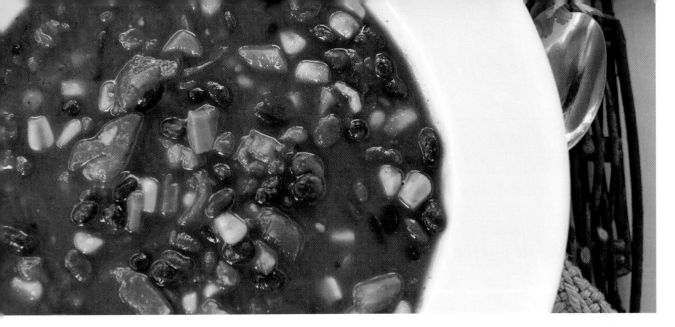

DAY 9

Cruciferous vegetables are not only the most powerful anti-cancer foods in existence; they are also the most micronutrient-dense of all vegetables. The cruciferous vegetables include: kale, collards, broccoli, cauliflower, cabbage and Brussels sprouts.

BREAKFAST

CHOCOLATE CHERRY SMOOTHIE
1 SERVING

3 cups chopped kale, tough stems removed

⅓ cup unsweetened, unflavored or vanilla soy, hemp or almond milk

⅓ cup pomegranate juice or ½ cup pomegranate kernels

1 tablespoon natural cocoa powder

1 cup frozen cherries

½ ripe banana *(peel and freeze the other half—you can use it to make healthy ice cream)*

Blend ingredients in a high-powered blender.

LUNCH

SALAD STUFFED PITA
1 SERVING

1 (100% whole grain) pita

4 avocado slices

2 tomato slices

1 cup shredded lettuce or spinach

2 onion slices

Russian Dressing *(from Day 7 lunch)*

Lightly toast the pita. Cut pita in half to form a pocket. Stuff with **Russian Dressing** and other ingredients.

Men: Add ¼ cup raw nuts and/or seeds

If you are following a gluten-free diet, skip the pita bread and make a big salad using additional greens and veggies.

Banana or other fruit for dessert

> **Tip:** When choosing a whole-grain bread, pita or wrap, read the ingredient list carefully to make sure it is 100% whole grain. It should list "whole" grain as the first ingredient. If more than one grain is used, they should all be whole grains. Just because a bread product claims to be multigrain or whole wheat, it does not mean it is 100% whole grain.

DINNER

BUENAS NOCHES BLACK BEAN SOUP
4 SERVINGS

1 small onion, chopped

1 cup chopped celery

1 cup chopped carrots

2 cloves garlic, chopped

2 teaspoons ground cumin

1 teaspoon chili powder

4 cups water

2 (15 ounce) cans low sodium black beans, drained, divided

1 cup low sodium salsa

1 cup frozen corn, thawed

1 cup diced tomatoes

In a large soup pot, combine onion, celery, carrots, garlic, cumin, chili powder, black pepper, water, and 2 cups of the beans. Bring to a boil, reduce heat and simmer for 15 minutes.

Place remaining black beans and the salsa in a blender or food processor. Blend on high speed until smooth. Stir into soup mixture along with the corn and tomatoes. Simmer for an additional 15 minutes.

Men: Have an extra serving of soup

Refrigerate leftover soup or freeze in individual portions and use for a quick and easy alternate lunch or dinner.

Serve with your choice of cooked vegetable (at least 2 cups cooked)

DAY 10

Achieve permanent weight control and superior health by eating more nutrient-rich foods and fewer high-calorie, low-nutrient foods. The more high-nutrient foods you consume, the fewer low-nutrient foods you desire.

BREAKFAST

BLUEBERRY BREAKFAST COBBLER
1 SERVING

½ banana, sliced
½ cup fresh or frozen blueberries
2 tablespoons uncooked old fashioned rolled oats
1 tablespoon raisins or currants
2 tablespoons chopped raw almonds
1 tablespoon unsweetened, shredded coconut
¼ teaspoon cinnamon

Combine banana, berries, oats and raisins in a microwave-safe dish. Microwave for 2 minutes. Top with almonds, cinnamon and coconut and microwave for 1 minute. Serve warm.

Men: Double the recipe

Tip: Season your foods with fresh or dried herbs and spices instead of salt. Experiment with a wide variety of seasoning options and soon you will not even miss the salt.

LUNCH

JAMAICAN JERK VEGETABLE SALAD
2 SERVINGS

¼ teaspoon dried thyme
¼ teaspoon garlic powder
¼ teaspoon dried cinnamon
¼ teaspoon ground allspice
⅛ teaspoon ground black pepper
⅛ teaspoon ground red cayenne pepper
1 cup sliced zucchini
1 small onion, cut into ⅛ inch slices
1 cup sliced red bell pepper
2 Portobello mushrooms, cut into ¼ inch slices
1 teaspoon rice vinegar
2 teaspoons lime juice
½ cup cooked black beans
1 mango, peeled and diced, divided
5 ounces mixed baby greens

Combine first six ingredients in a large zip lock plastic bag. Add zucchini, onion, bell pepper, mushrooms, vinegar and lime juice. Seal and shake well to coat.

Lightly wipe a large nonstick skillet with oil. Add vegetable mixture and sauté for 5 minutes or until vegetables are tender, adding a small amount of water if necessary to prevent sticking. Add black beans, ½ cup of the chopped mango and continue cooking for another 2 minutes. Remove from heat.

Serve vegetables on a bed of mixed greens, topped with remaining diced mango.

Men: Add one cup of beans to the salad

DINNER

VEGGIES AND ORANGE PEANUT DIP
(leftover from Day 8 dinner)

SZECHUAN SESAME STIR FRY
2 SERVINGS

For the Sauce:
2 tablespoons unhulled sesame seeds, lightly toasted
½ cup unsweetened non-dairy milk
4 dates, pitted
1 teaspoon minced ginger
1 clove garlic, peeled
⅛ teaspoon red pepper flakes, or to taste
1 ½ tablespoons rice vinegar

For the Stir Fry:
1 cup broccoli florets
1 cup cauliflower florets
½ red bell pepper, cut into 1 inch pieces
1 cup sliced shiitake mushrooms
½ cup snow peas
2 cups cooked wild rice or quinoa
2 ounces cooked shredded chicken, optional

In a high-powered blender, puree all of the sauce ingredients until smooth. Set aside.

Heat ¼ cup of water in a wok or large sauté pan. Add broccoli and cauliflower, cover and steam for 6 minutes. Remove cover and add bell pepper, mushrooms and snow peas and stir fry for an additional 5 minutes or until vegetables are crisp-tender. Add small amounts of water as needed to prevent sticking.

Add sesame sauce to veggies and continue to stir fry for 1-2 minutes to heat through. Serve over rice or quinoa. Top with chicken if desired.

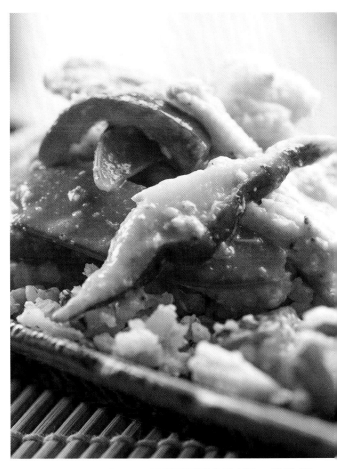

DAYS 11-15
SHOPPING LIST

This shopping list assumes that all recipes in the meal plan will be made. Menus frequently include fruit for dessert and will mention a specific fruit as an example. That fruit is used for the shopping list.

Check your refrigerator, freezer and pantry before shopping. You may have items leftover from Days 1-10 that you can use. Make sure you also have all the items listed in the Stock Your Pantry list.

FRESH PRODUCE
VEGETABLES

- [ ] 2 heads romaine lettuce
- [ ] 5 cups mixed greens (about 5 ounces)
- [ ] 2 bunches (3 for men) kale
- [ ] 14 ounces spinach (10 ounces could be frozen)
- [ ] Your choice of a green vegetable to equal 2 cups cooked (could also buy frozen)
- [ ] 2-3 broccoli crowns (need at least 2 cups after cooking)
- [ ] Red cabbage (any leftovers? Need 2 cups shredded)
- [ ] 1 large eggplant
- [ ] 2 medium tomatoes
- [ ] Pint cherry tomatoes (need 6)
- [ ] Small package edamame in the pod (could also buy frozen)
- [ ] 2 avocados
- [ ] 1 red bell pepper
- [ ] 2 green bell peppers
- [ ] Poblano chili pepper, optional (see Day 11 dinner)
- [ ] 1 cucumber
- [ ] 1 mushroom
- [ ] 4 ounces white or cremini mushroom

- [ ] 2 carrots
- [ ] 1 stalk celery
- [ ] 2 red onions
- [ ] 5 yellow onions
- [ ] 1 head garlic
- [ ] Cilantro
- [ ] Basil
- [ ] Add 1 small butternut squash for men (need 2 cups chopped, could also buy frozen)

FRUIT

- [ ] 2 pints (about 4 cups) blueberries (or 20 ounces of frozen)
- [ ] 1 pound strawberries (could also buy frozen)
- [ ] 2 (4 for men) bananas
- [ ] 6 apples
- [ ] Small bunch of grapes
- [ ] 1 cantaloupe or honeydew melon
- [ ] 2 lemons

REFRIGERATED

- [ ] ¾ cup (1 ½ cups for men) pomegranate juice
- [ ] Small package non-dairy mozzarella-type cheese (need ⅓ cup shredded) Any left from Days 1-10?

- [ ] 2 cups (3 cups for men) unsweetened soy, hemp or almond milk. You can use all unflavored or if desired, use vanilla unsweetened for breakfast and smoothie recipes and unflavored unsweetened for other recipes. You will need about 1 ¼ cups vanilla (2 ¼ cups for men) and ⅔ cup unflavored non-dairy milk.

FROZEN

This list does not include foods that have a frozen option on the Fresh Produce list. Check to see what you have left over from Days 1-10

- [ ] 16 ounces (need 3 ⅓ cups) frozen corn
- [ ] 10 ounces (need 1 cup) frozen broccoli
- [ ] 16-20 ounces (women need 2 cups; men need 3) frozen blueberries
- [ ] Add 1 cup of frozen cherries for men

SHELF STABLE
BEANS

It is assumed that canned, low sodium or no-salt-added beans will be used. If you opt to start with dry beans, 1 cup of dry beans will yield about 3 cups of cooked beans

- [ ] 1 (15-ounce) can black beans
- [ ] 1 (15-ounce) can chickpeas
- [ ] 3 (15-ounce) cans red kidney beans
- [ ] Dry lentils (need 1 cup)

OTHER

Choose tomato products packaged in cartons or glass. These materials do not contain BPA.

- [ ] Low sodium or no-salt-added vegetable juice or carrot juice (need ½ cup)
- [ ] Low sodium tomato sauce (need 1 cup)
- [ ] Low sodium diced tomatoes (need 38 ounces)
- [ ] Low sodium pasta sauce (need 2 ½ cups)
- [ ] Low sodium salsa (need ¼ cup)

DAY 11

Eating for optimal health and weight loss is not about deprivation. It is about consuming large quantities of foods which have a high nutrient-to-calorie ratio.

BREAKFAST

BERRY BOWL
1 SERVING

1 ½ cups blueberries, strawberries, blackberries and/or raspberries
1 banana, sliced
¼ cup unsweetened, unflavored or vanilla soy, hemp or almond milk
2 tablespoons chopped walnuts
1 tablespoon ground flax or chia seeds

Top berries and banana with non-dairy milk and sprinkle with the walnuts and flax or chia seeds.

Men: Increase chopped walnuts to ¼ cup.

LUNCH

SWEET KALE SALAD
1 SERVING

5 cups chopped kale, tough stems and center ribs removed
1 tablespoon lemon juice
1 small apple, cored and sliced
1 tablespoon raw sunflower seeds or pumpkin seeds
1 tablespoon raisins
½ avocado, peeled and chopped
Balsamic or fig-flavored vinegar

Toss together all ingredients except vinegar. Finish with a splash of vinegar.

(Wrap up the leftover avocado, refrigerate and save for tomorrow)

Grapes or other fruit for dessert

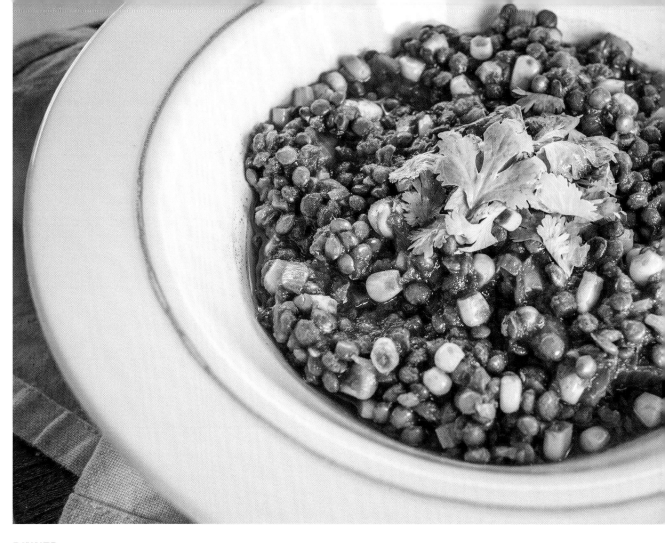

DINNER

LAZY LENTILS
4 SERVINGS

1 cup dry lentils
1 cup frozen corn
1 cup low sodium tomato sauce
1 medium onion, chopped
½ teaspoon cumin powder
1 teaspoon chili powder
2 tablespoons fresh cilantro
Poblano chili peppers, optional

Boil the lentils in 2 cups of water for 30 minutes or until tender and then drain. Stir in the corn, tomato sauce, onion, cumin and chili powder and simmer over low heat for 20 minutes. Stir in cilantro.

If desired, serve lentils in halved Poblano chili peppers.

Men: Add 2 cups cooked butternut squash to the lentils

Quick and easy lunch option for tomorrow: Leftover Lazy Lentils on a bed of baby greens

Serve with steamed or water-sautéed broccoli or other vegetable

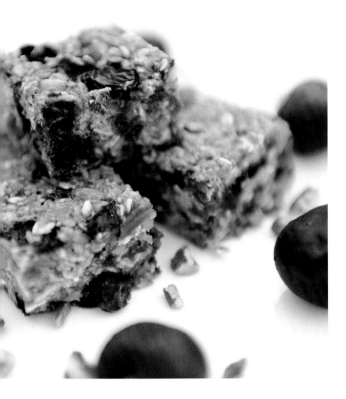

DAY 12

The most important building block of health is nutrition. Without superior nutrition, your ability to live life to the fullest is limited. Unfortunately, most of modern society lives on a low-nutrient diet of empty-calorie, processed, refined foods.

BREAKFAST

ANTIOXIDANT-RICH BREAKFAST BARS
6 SERVINGS

1 medium ripe banana
1 cup old fashioned oats
1 cup frozen blueberries, thawed
¼ cup raisins
⅛ cup pomegranate juice
2 tablespoons finely chopped dates
2 tablespoons chopped walnuts
2 tablespoons ground flax seed

Mash banana in a large bowl. Add remaining ingredients and mix thoroughly. Spread mixture into an 8-inch square baking pan that has been lightly wiped with olive oil. Bake for 25 minutes at 350 degrees F. Cool on wire rack and cut into bars.

Refrigerate or freeze leftover bars and use them as an alternate breakfast. **Limit -1 per day**

Men: Add a green smoothie. Try the Eat your Greens Smoothie (see Day 13)

LUNCH

MEXICAN SALAD *(or leftover Lazy Lentils from last night on a bed of greens)*
1 SERVING

1 head romaine lettuce, chopped
⅓ cup cooked black beans
⅓ cup frozen, thawed corn kernels
¼ cup low sodium salsa
½ avocado, peeled and chopped

Toss lettuce with beans, corn and salsa. Top your salad with the chopped avocado.

Save leftover black beans for later in the week

Apple or other fruit for dessert

Men: Spread 2 tablespoons almond or cashew butter on apple slices or have ¼ cup raw nuts and/or seeds

DINNER

EASY VEGETABLE PIZZA
1 SERVING

1 large (100% whole grain) tortilla
½ cup low sodium pasta sauce
¼ cup chopped mushrooms
¼ cup chopped red onion
1 cup frozen broccoli, thawed and chopped
1 tablespoon shredded non-dairy mozzarella-type cheese, optional

Preheat oven to 200 degrees F. Place tortilla on a baking sheet and warm for 10 minutes. Remove from oven and top with remaining ingredients. Bake for 30 minutes.

If you are following a gluten-free diet, substitute a dinner item from another night.

Your choice of a steamed or water-sautéed green vegetable or a mixed green salad with tomatoes, onions and other veggies and Healthy Caesar Dressing

> **Tip:** Steaming a veggie is quick and easy. You only need a steamer pot with a lid or a steamer basket to place in a pot with a lid. Add a small amount of water, cover and cook until the vegetables have just started to become tender but still retain some firmness.

HEALTHY CAESAR DRESSING
4 SERVINGS

4 cloves garlic or ¼ teaspoon garlic powder
⅔ cup unsweetened soy, almond or hemp milk
⅓ cup raw cashew butter or ⅔ cup raw cashews
1 ½ tablespoons nutritional yeast
1 tablespoon plus 1 teaspoon fresh lemon juice
2 teaspoons Dijon mustard
dash black pepper

If using fresh garlic, roast in a 350 degree F oven for about 25 minutes or until soft. Cool and remove skins.

Blend roasted garlic (or garlic powder) with the remaining ingredients in a high-powered blender until creamy and smooth. If using cashew butter, ingredients can also be whisked together instead of using a blender.

Save leftover dressing for another meal. If you are pressed for time and opt for a bottled dressing, use a no-oil dressing that contains no more than 75 mg of sodium per tablespoon and add 1-2 tablespoons of raw nuts or seeds to enhance the absorption of nutrients from the salad.

DAY 13

The quality of the food is what makes the dish. The simplest ingredients are delicious as long as they are top quality. Don't skimp on quality or freshness.

BREAKFAST

EAT YOUR GREENS FRUIT SMOOTHIE
1 SERVING

2 cups kale or other greens

½ banana (freeze the other half—frozen bananas are great for smoothies and healthy desserts)

1 cup frozen or fresh blueberries

½ cup unsweetened, unflavored or vanilla soy, hemp or almond milk

½ cup pomegranate juice

1 tablespoon ground flaxseeds

Blend all ingredients in a high-powered blender until smooth and creamy.

Men: Add a leftover Antioxidant-Rich Breakfast Bar from Day 12

LUNCH

PITA STUFFED WITH SEASONED GREENS
1 SERVING

5-6 large leaves kale, Swiss chard or mustard greens, tough stems removed

1 teaspoon lemon juice

1 (100% whole grain) pita

dash garlic powder

2 thin slices red onion

sliced tomato

Dijon mustard

Steam the greens until tender, about 10-15 minutes. Sprinkle with lemon juice and garlic powder.

Stuff whole-grain pita with greens, red onion and tomato. Add mustard if desired.

Men: Add hummus or sliced avocado

If you are following a gluten-free diet, have the greens with a baked sweet potato.

Serve with edamame sprinkled with salt-free seasoning

Fresh or thawed frozen berries for dessert

DINNER

MIXED GREENS SALAD WITH TOMATOES, ONIONS, SHREDDED RED CABBAGE AND HEALTHY CAESAR DRESSING *(see Day 12 dinner) or bottled no-oil, low sodium dressing*

EGGPLANT ROLL UPS
3 SERVINGS

1 large eggplant, peeled and sliced lengthwise ¼ inch thick

2-3 tablespoons water

1 medium red bell pepper, seeded and coarsely chopped

1 small onion, coarsely chopped

½ cup chopped carrots

¼ cup chopped celery

2 cloves garlic, chopped

4 ounces baby spinach

1 teaspoon no-salt seasoning blend, such as Mrs. Dash adjusted to taste

2 cups no-salt-added or low sodium pasta sauce, divided

¼ cup shredded non-dairy mozzarella-type cheese, optional

Preheat oven to 350 degrees F. Arrange eggplant in a single layer on a lightly-oiled baking pan. Bake about 20 minutes or until eggplant is flexible enough to roll up easily.

Meanwhile, heat 2 tablespoons water in a large pan, add the bell pepper, onion, carrots, celery, and garlic; sauté until just tender, adding more water if needed. Add the spinach and no-salt seasoning and cook until spinach is wilted. Transfer to a mixing bowl and mix in 3 tablespoons of the pasta sauce and the shredded cheese.

Spread about ¼ cup of the pasta sauce in the bottom of a baking pan. Put some of the vegetable mixture on each eggplant slice, roll up and place in a pan. Pour the remaining sauce over the eggplant rolls. Bake for 20-30 minutes, until heated through.

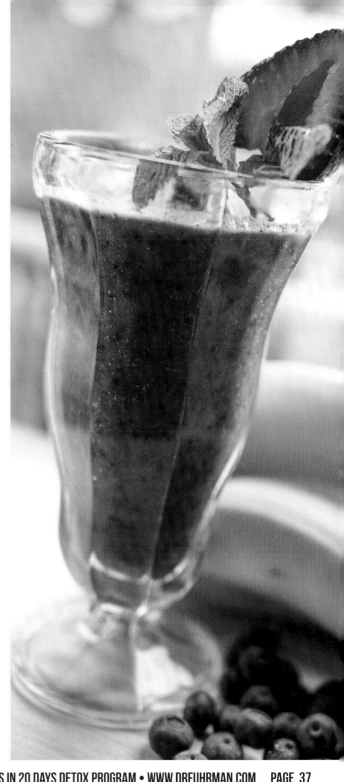

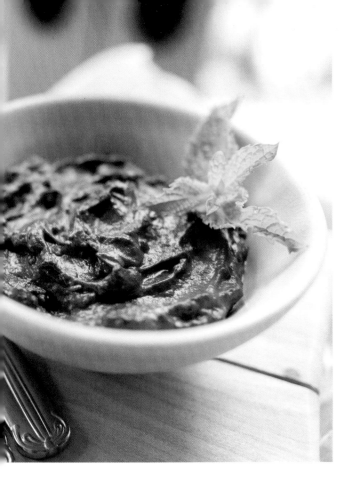

DAY 14

Nutrient-rich foods such as fresh vegetables, fruit, beans, intact whole grains, raw nuts and seeds comprise only 13% of the calories in the standard American diet. This is alarming because a diet centered on milk, cheese, pasta, bread, fried foods, and sugar-filled snacks and drinks lays the groundwork for obesity, cancer, heart disease and diabetes.

BREAKFAST

CHIA SEED BREAKFAST PUDDING
1 SERVING

½ cup unsweetened, unflavored or vanilla soy, hemp or almond milk

2 tablespoons whole chia seeds

2 tablespoons uncooked old fashioned oats

½ banana, sliced (peel and freeze the other half—you will use it to make a healthy ice cream)

½ cup fresh blueberries or frozen, thawed

In a bowl, mix together non-dairy milk, chia seeds and oats. Let mixture sit for 10 minutes or, for an on-the-run breakfast, make the night before and refrigerate. Stir in banana and blueberries.

Men: Add the Chocolate Cherry Smoothie (see Day 9)

LUNCH

BIG GREEN SALAD WITH EASY BALSAMIC ALMOND DRESSING

Include tomatoes, red onions, shredded red cabbage, other veggies and ½ cup cooked or canned low sodium chickpeas or other beans

EASY BALSAMIC ALMOND DRESSING
1 SERVING

2 tablespoons water

1 tablespoon plus 1 teaspoon balsamic vinegar

1 tablespoon raw almond butter

¼ teaspoon onion powder

¼ teaspoon garlic powder

⅛ teaspoon dried oregano

⅛ teaspoon dried basil

Whisk water, vinegar and almond butter together until mixture is smooth and almond butter is evenly dispersed. Mix in remaining ingredients.

Melon or other fruit for dessert

DINNER

TAILGATE CHILI
5 SERVINGS

If you made this on Day 3, you may have some left in the freezer.

½ cup uncooked bulgur or quinoa

1 cup water

3 cups chopped onions

3 cloves garlic, minced

2 green bell peppers, chopped

26 ounces low sodium diced tomatoes (see note)

3 (15 ounce) cans red kidney beans, no salt added or low sodium, rinsed and drained

2 cups fresh or frozen corn kernels

2 tablespoons chili powder

2 teaspoons ground cumin

Combine bulgur or quinoa and water in a saucepan. Bring to a boil, reduce heat and simmer for 12 to 15 minutes or until tender.

Meanwhile, heat ⅛ cup water in a large saucepan and water sauté onions and garlic until almost soft, about 5 minutes. Stir in green peppers and sauté an additional 3 minutes, adding more water as needed. Stir in diced tomatoes, beans, corn, chili powder and cumin. Bring to a boil, reduce heat, cover and simmer for 20 minutes. Add bulgur or quinoa and simmer for an additional 5 minutes.

Note: Choose tomato products packaged in cartons or glass. These materials do not contain BPA.

Men: Have an extra serving of chili

Portion leftover chili into individual containers. If you like, you can have another serving tomorrow for lunch. Use the remaining servings for alternate lunches or dinners over the next 3-4 days if you are short on time, or freeze for later use.

AVOCADO CHOCOLATE PUDDING
4 SERVINGS

1 ripe avocado, peeled, pit removed

½ to ¾ cups water (start with a ½ cup and add more if needed to blend)

4 tablespoons natural non-alkalized cocoa powder

6 regular dates, pitted

dash vanilla extract

Blend all ingredients in a high-powered blender.

Enjoy this chocolaty pudding by itself tonight, and then over the next few days, try it as a topping for fresh fruit.

DAY 15

A key step to achieving dietary excellence, attaining ideal weight and enjoying excellent health is getting rid of your food addictions. It only takes a few seconds of decision making to say an emphatic no to the addiction, and yes to your new, healthful diet and lifestyle.

BREAKFAST

APPLE SURPRISE
SERVES 3

½ cup raisins
¼ cup water
4 apples, peeled, cored and diced
¼ cup chopped walnuts
2 tablespoons ground flax seeds
½ tablespoon cinnamon

Place raisins in bottom of pot and cover with ¼ cup water.

Place diced apples on top. Cover and steam over very low heat for 7 minutes.

Transfer apple/raisin mixture to a bowl and mix well with remaining ingredients.

Men: Have 2 servings of Apple Surprise

This recipe keeps well in the refrigerator for several days so you can have it as an alternate breakfast or even a dessert.

LUNCH

PORTOBELLO SALAD WITH LEMON BASIL VINAIGRETTE
SALAD: 1 SERVING; DRESSING: 4 SERVINGS

1 Portobello mushroom
5 cups mixed greens
¼ cup sliced red onion

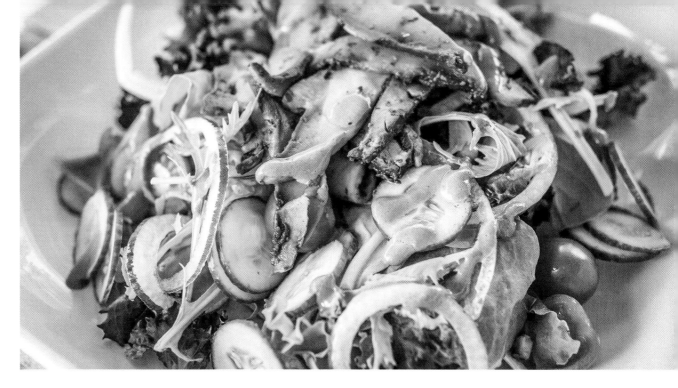

½ cucumber, sliced
6 cherry tomatoes

For the Lemon Basil Vinaigrette:
2 tablespoons fresh lemon juice
2 tablespoons balsamic vinegar
½ cup water
¼ cup raw almonds or ⅛ cup raw almond butter
¼ cup raisins
⅓ cup fresh basil leaves
1 teaspoon Dijon mustard
1 clove garlic

Slice the Portobello mushroom and sauté in water, vegetable broth or white wine (or grill it). Toss together baby greens, onion, cucumber and tomatoes. Top with the sliced mushroom.

For the dressing, combine all ingredients in a high-powered blender. Drizzle desired amount of dressing over salad.

Store the remaining dressing in the fridge; you can use it on your salad on Day 18.

Men: Have some leftover soup or chili

Melon or other fruit for dessert

DINNER

CHICKPEA CURRY IN A HURRY
2 SERVINGS

1 ½ cups (a 15-ounce can) cooked chickpeas
½ cup low sodium vegetable broth
1 ½ cups diced tomatoes
1 teaspoon garlic powder
2 teaspoons curry powder
⅓ cup unsweetened dried coconut
1 10-ounce box or bag frozen chopped spinach

Combine all ingredients except spinach in a large saucepan. Cook for 5 minutes, then add spinach. Cover and continue cooking until spinach is thawed and curry is warm, about 5 more minutes. Serve over quinoa or other whole grain.

Enjoy one serving tonight and save one for lunch tomorrow or another time when you are too busy to cook.

Serve with 1 cup of quinoa, farro or other intact whole grain

Fresh or thawed frozen berries for dessert

DAYS 16-20
SHOPPING LIST

This shopping list assumes that all recipes in the meal plan will be made. Menus frequently include fruit for dessert and will mention a specific fruit as an example. That fruit is used for the shopping list.

Check your refrigerator, freezer and pantry before shopping. You may have items leftover from Days 1-15 that you can use. Make sure you also have all the items listed in the Stock Your Pantry list.

FRESH PRODUCE

VEGETABLES

- [ ] 3 heads romaine lettuce
- [ ] 8 cups mixed greens (about 8 ounces)
- [ ] 2 bunches kale
- [ ] 5 ounces spinach
- [ ] Your choice of a green vegetable to equal 2 cups cooked (could also buy frozen)
- [ ] Red cabbage (any leftover? Need 1 cup shredded)
- [ ] 3 medium tomatoes
- [ ] 6 plum tomatoes
- [ ] 1 (2 for men) avocado
- [ ] 3 zucchini
- [ ] 3 red peppers
- [ ] 1 Poblano chili pepper
- [ ] 2 Portobello mushrooms
- [ ] 15 ounces white or cremini mushrooms

- [ ] 1 sweet potato
- [ ] 2 carrots
- [ ] 2 red onions
- [ ] 5 yellow onions
- [ ] 4 green onions (scallions)
- [ ] 1 head garlic
- [ ] Cilantro
- [ ] Basil
- [ ] Tarragon (could also use dried tarragon)

FRUIT

- [ ] 1 pound strawberries
- [ ] 2 bananas
- [ ] Small bunch of grapes
- [ ] Cantaloupe or honeydew melon
- [ ] 2 mangos
- [ ] 3 lemons
- [ ] 2 limes

REFRIGERATED

- [ ] 1 ½ cups unsweetened, unflavored or vanilla soy, hemp or almond milk
- [ ] ⅓ cup pomegranate juice
- [ ] 7 ounces extra firm tofu
- [ ] 1 egg, optional
- [ ] ½ cup shredded cooked organic chicken breast, optional
- [ ] 4 ounces ground organic turkey (for vegan black bean burgers, purchase an additional 15 ounce can of black beans)

FROZEN

This list does not include foods that have a frozen option listed on the Fresh Produce list. Check to see what you have left over from Days 1-15.

- [ ] ½ cup frozen corn (any leftover?)
- [ ] 10 ounces frozen blueberries
- [ ] 10 ounces frozen strawberries
- [ ] 12 ounces frozen cherries
- [ ] 10 ounces frozen mango

SHELF STABLE

BEANS

It is assumed that canned, low sodium or no-salt-added beans will be used. If you opt to start with dry beans, 1 cup of dry beans will yield about 3 cups of cooked beans.

- [ ] 2 (15 ounce) cans black beans
- [ ] 2 (15 ounce) cans cannellini or other white beans
- [ ] 2 (15 ounce) cans chickpeas
- [ ] 2 (15 ounce) cans pinto beans
- [ ] 1 (15 ounce) can any variety beans

OTHER

Choose tomato products packaged in cartons or glass. These materials do not contain BPA.

- [ ] Low sodium or no-salt-added vegetable broth (need 5 cups)
- [ ] Low sodium diced tomatoes (need 30 ounces)
- [ ] Low sodium salsa (need ½ cup)

DAY 16

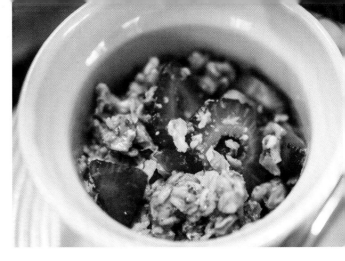

Eating a large amount of greens and other colorful vegetables is the secret to achieving great health and your ideal body weight. These vegetables are low in calories and high in life-extending nutrients. Eat these foods in unlimited quantities and think big. Try to eat a pound of raw vegetables and a pound of cooked vegetables each day. If you can't eat this much, don't force yourself—but the idea is to completely rethink what constitutes a portion.

BREAKFAST

NO-COOK STRAWBERRY OATMEAL TO GO
1 SERVING

⅓ cup uncooked old fashioned oats
1 tablespoon chia seeds
⅔ cup unsweetened, unflavored or vanilla soy, hemp or almond milk
1 cup fresh or thawed frozen strawberries, sliced (or blueberries, cherries or sliced peaches)
6 walnut halves, crushed

Place the oats and chia seeds in a portable cup, add non-dairy milk and refrigerate overnight. In the morning, stir in sliced strawberries and walnuts.

Men: Increase walnuts to ¼ cup

LUNCH

BLACK BEAN MANGO SALAD
2 SERVINGS

½ cup frozen corn, thawed
1 mango, peeled, pitted and cubed
1 tablespoon chopped fresh cilantro
2 green onions, thinly sliced
½ medium red bell pepper, seeded and chopped
1 ½ cups cooked black beans or 1 (15 ounce) can no- or low-salt black beans drained and rinsed
1 ½ tablespoons fresh lime juice
½ teaspoon minced fresh garlic

½ teaspoon dried oregano
½ teaspoon ground cumin
dash chili powder
6 cups chopped romaine lettuce

Mix all the ingredients, except the lettuce in a bowl. Let stand for at least 15 minutes, then serve on top of the lettuce.

Leftover Black Bean Mango Salad can be enjoyed for lunch tomorrow.

> **Tip:** If you are pressed for time, you can use store-bought frozen veggie burgers. Select a product that does not contain isolated soy protein and is labeled low sodium or light in sodium.

DINNER

TURKEY BURGERS WITH BLACK BEANS AND MUSHROOMS
4 SERVINGS
(Vegan option: Black Bean and Mushroom Burgers)

1 cup chopped mushrooms
¼ cup old fashioned rolled oats
2 tablespoons raw pumpkin seeds
1 carrot, grated
1 cup cooked or canned low sodium black beans, drained
¼ teaspoon cumin
¼ teaspoon chili powder
¼ teaspoon onion powder

⅛ teaspoon black pepper
4 ounces ground organic turkey (For vegan burgers, omit turkey and use an additional cup of beans)

Preheat oven to 300 degrees F.

Heat 1-2 tablespoons water in a small pan and sauté mushrooms until tender and moisture has evaporated, about 5 minutes. Set aside.

Grind oats and pumpkin seeds in a food processor. Add grated carrots, ¾ cup of the beans (1 ¾ cups for vegan burgers) and all of the spices and process until blended.

Spoon mixture into a mixing bowl and stir in sautéed mushrooms, remaining ¼ cup whole beans and ground turkey. Form into 4 medium-sized patties. Place on a baking sheet lined with parchment paper or lightly wiped with olive oil. Bake for 40 minutes, turning once after 20 minutes.

Serve on a bed of mixed greens with sliced red onion and tomato or on a small 100% whole grain roll or pita with onion, tomato and lettuce.

Men: Add ½ avocado, sliced, and an extra burger without the roll.

Refrigerate or freeze leftover patties for another meal or enjoy your burgers with a friend.

Melon or other fruit for dessert

> **Tip:** Avoid packaged foods that contain more milligrams (mg) of sodium than the number of calories.

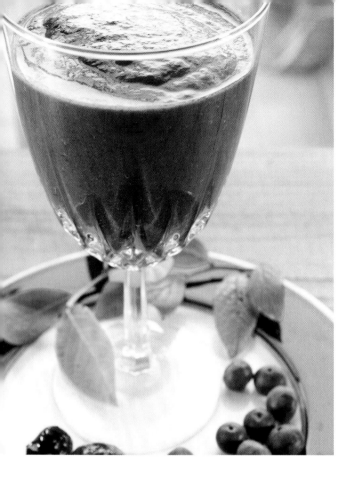

DAY 17

As you begin to eat healthful, nutrient-dense foods, you flood your body with the vitamins, minerals and phytochemicals it so desperately needs. You truly satisfy your hunger for perhaps the first time in your life.

BREAKFAST

CHOCOLATE CHERRY SMOOTHIE
1 SERVING

3 cups chopped kale, tough stems removed

⅓ cup unsweetened, unflavored or vanilla soy, hemp or almond milk

⅓ cup pomegranate juice

1 tablespoon natural cocoa powder

1 cup frozen cherries

½ ripe banana *(peel and freeze the other half—you can use it to make smoothies or healthy ice cream)*

Blend ingredients in a high-powered blender.

Men: Add 1 cup cooked steel cut or old fashioned oats with non-dairy milk and 1 cup fresh or thawed frozen fruit.

LUNCH

QUINOA BEAN SALAD
(or leftovers from one of the dinners you've made this week)
3 SERVINGS

1 cup cooked quinoa

1 cup cooked white beans or canned low sodium white beans

¼ cup dried raisins or currants

¼ cup walnuts, chopped

2 plum tomatoes, chopped

¼ cup chopped red onion

½ red bell pepper, chopped

1 teaspoon chili powder or more to taste

1 teaspoon Bragg Liquid Aminos or low sodium soy sauce

Place all ingredients in a large bowl and mix.

Grapes or other fruit for dessert

DINNER

QUICK GREENS AND WHITE BEAN STEW
3 SERVINGS

5 cups chopped kale or other greens, tough stems removed and coarsely chopped

¼ cup water

1 small onion, chopped

2 cloves garlic, minced

1 teaspoon no-salt seasoning blend, adjusted to taste

¼ teaspoon ground black pepper

⅛ teaspoon crushed red pepper or to taste

1 ½ cups cooked cannellini or other white beans or 1 (15 ounce) can low sodium or no-salt-added, drained

15 ounces (1 ½ cups) diced tomatoes

3 cups low sodium vegetable broth, or more if needed to achieve desired consistency

Add kale and water to a soup pot, cover and cook over medium heat for 10 minutes or until kale is tender, stirring occasionally.

Add onion, garlic, no-salt seasoning, black pepper and red pepper. Continue to cook, uncovered, for 5-7 more minutes.

Add beans, tomatoes and vegetable broth and bring to boil.

Reduce heat and simmer, covered for 15-20 minutes, stirring occasionally.

Men: Have an extra serving of soup

Refrigerate leftover soup or freeze in individual portions to enjoy as an alternative lunch or dinner.

CRISPY KALE CHIPS
3 SERVINGS

1 small bunch kale, tough stems and center ribs removed, torn into uniform pieces

Choice of Seasonings:
garlic and/or onion powder
Dr. Fuhrman's VegiZest or MatoZest
Mrs. Dash no-salt seasoning blends
chili powder and cumin

Preheat oven to 350 degrees F. Spread kale evenly on a non-stick baking sheet which has been lined with parchment paper or lightly wiped with olive oil.

Sprinkle with your choice of seasoning. Bake for 10 to 15 minutes or until crispy and dry, tossing occasionally to prevent burning.

DAY 18

Foods of animal origin are high in calories and very low in nutrients per calorie, compared to vegetables. It is best to restrict animal-source products (meat, dairy and eggs) to two or fewer servings per week and only one or two ounces at a time.

BREAKFAST

TOFU SCRAMBLE (WITH OPTIONAL EGG)
1 SERVING

2 scallions, diced
¼ cup finely chopped red bell pepper
1 small tomato, chopped
1 clove garlic, minced or pressed
7 ounces extra firm tofu, drained and crumbled (reduce to 3½ ounces if using egg)
1 egg, beaten, optional
½ teaspoon no-salt seasoning blend such as Mrs. Dash
1 tablespoon nutritional yeast
3 cups coarsely chopped spinach

Sauté scallions, red pepper, tomato, and garlic in ¼ cup water for 5 minutes. Add tofu, egg if desired, no-salt seasoning blend, nutritional yeast and spinach, and cook for another 2 minutes.

May be served with low sodium ketchup or salsa. For some heat, add some hot pepper flakes.

Men: Add 2 cups of fresh or thawed frozen fruit topped with flax, hemp or chia seeds

LUNCH

BIG GREEN SALAD WITH LEMON BASIL VINAIGRETTE

Include tomatoes, red onions, shredded red cabbage, other veggies and ½ cup of cooked or canned low sodium black, white or red beans

Men: Increase beans to 1 cup and add ½ avocado, sliced

LEMON BASIL VINAIGRETTE *(Left over from Day 15)*
4 SERVINGS

2 tablespoons fresh lemon juice
2 tablespoons balsamic vinegar
½ cup water
¼ cup raw almonds or ⅛ cup raw almond butter
¼ cup raisins
⅓ cup fresh basil leaves
1 teaspoon Dijon mustard
1 clove garlic

Combine all ingredients in a high-powered blender.

Thawed frozen cherries or other fruit for dessert

DINNER

MUSHROOM STROGANOFF
2 SERVINGS

1 medium onion, chopped
2 cloves garlic, minced
10 ounces mushrooms, thinly sliced
2 tablespoons fresh lemon juice
1 tablespoon fresh tarragon, chopped or 1 teaspoon dried tarragon
1 tablespoon sweet paprika
1 cup no-salt-added or low sodium vegetable broth
3 tablespoons unhulled sesame seeds pureed with ¼ cup water

In a nonstick skillet, water sauté onion and garlic until soft. Add mushrooms and continue cooking until mushrooms soften and lose their moisture. Add lemon juice, tarragon and paprika and mix well.

Whisk together vegetable broth and pureed sesame seeds. (Heating the broth makes blending easier.)

Pour over mushroom mixture and mix well. Simmer until mixture thickens slightly or until desired consistency.

Serve with wild rice or steamed kale or spinach.

> **Tip:** It is easy to shop for nutrient-dense foods. They are found mostly in the produce aisle.

STRAWBEANY ICE CREAM
4 SERVINGS

1 cup frozen strawberries
¾ cup cooked pinto beans
6 regular dates or 3 Medjool dates, pitted
½ cup raw cashews
1 teaspoon vanilla extract
2 ½ cups water
½ cup sliced fresh organic strawberries

Blend dates, frozen strawberries, cashews, beans, vanilla, and water in a high-powered blender until well blended. Pour into a bowl. Stir in ½ cup sliced fresh strawberries.

Freeze until almost set, about 2-4 hours.

Portion leftover ice cream into individual servings and freeze. Enjoy with another meal.

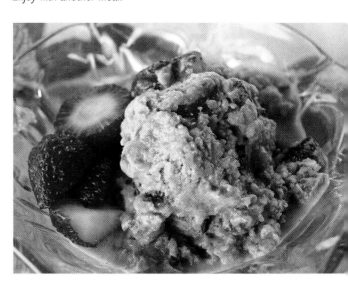

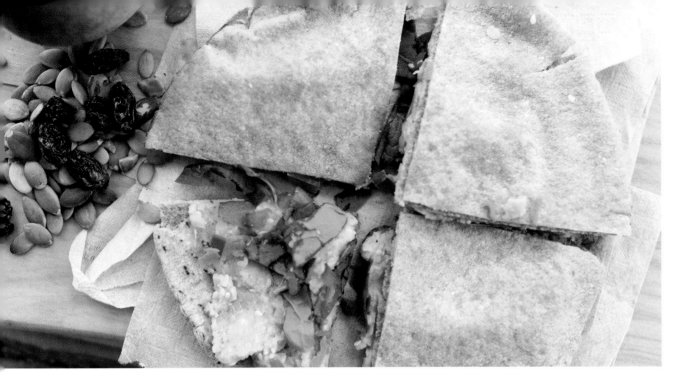

DAY 19

A high-nutrient diet will reduce your desire for high-calorie, low-nutrient foods. Your taste buds will change and you'll lose interest in the unhealthy foods you once thought you could never live without. You'll feel more satisfied eating fewer calories than you were eating before.

BREAKFAST

BLENDED MANGO SALAD
1 SERVING

1 ½ cups frozen mango chunks

2 cups spinach

1 cup chopped romaine lettuce

¼ cup unsweetened, unflavored or vanilla non-dairy milk or coconut water

½ tablespoon ground flax seeds

Blend ingredients in a high-powered blender or food processor

Men: Add Banana and Nut Butter Lettuce Wraps:

2 tablespoons raw cashew or almond butter

6 romaine lettuce leaves

1 banana, sliced

Spread about 1 teaspoon nut butter on each lettuce leaf. Lay a few banana slices on top and roll up like a burrito.

LUNCH

HUMMUS AND RED PEPPER PITA TRIANGLES
1 SERVING

¼ cup hummus (see recipe from Day 3 lunch)

1 (100% whole grain) pita, split in half crosswise

¼ cup red bell pepper, finely chopped

1 small carrot, grated

1 cup baby spinach leaves, or lettuce

Spread pita halves with hummus and top with chopped red pepper, grated carrot, spinach and the other half of the pita. Cut into quarters.

You can also make wraps using whole-grain tortillas.

Men: Have an additional ¼ cup hummus with assorted raw veggies and ¼ cup raw nuts and/or seeds.

For a gluten-free option, have hummus with lots of raw veggies and add a salad or perhaps leftovers from earlier in the week.

Fresh or thawed frozen berries for dessert

DINNER

CHUNKY SWEET POTATO STEW
2 SERVINGS

1 onion, sliced

2 large garlic cloves, chopped

15 ounces (1 ½ cups) diced tomatoes

1 large sweet potato, peeled, cut into ½ inch pieces

1 cup cooked or no-salt-added or low sodium canned garbanzo beans (chickpeas) or white kidney beans

½ cup low sodium or no-salt-added vegetable broth

¾ teaspoon dried rosemary

1 medium zucchini, cut into ½ inch thick rounds

1 teaspoon Mrs. Dash or other no-salt seasoning

In a sauté pan, heat 2 tablespoons water, then add the onion and garlic and water sauté about 5 minutes, until slightly softened, separating the onion slices into rings. Add a little extra water if the pan gets too dry. Mix in tomatoes, sweet potato, garbanzo beans, vegetable broth and rosemary. Bring mixture to a simmer, stirring occasionally. Cover and cook 5 minutes, slightly mashing some of the garbanzo beans. Add zucchini. Cover and cook until sweet potato pieces are tender, about 15 minutes, stirring occasionally. Season with no-salt seasoning.

Add your choice of cooked green or other high-nutrient vegetable
The high-nutrient, non-green vegetables are: tomatoes, onions, mushrooms, cauliflower, eggplant and red peppers.

DAY 20

You have begun to see weight loss results, you feel better, your taste buds are more sensitive and you have made a good start at losing your cravings to overeat. Don't stop now! Don't go back to your old way of eating. Continue on your journey and make a permanent change in your eating habits. Not only will you reach your ideal weight—you will be rewarded with a lifetime of good health.

BREAKFAST

BLUEBERRY BREAKFAST COBBLER
1 SERVING

½ banana, sliced
½ cup frozen blueberries
2 tablespoons uncooked old fashioned rolled oats
1 tablespoon raisins or currants
2 tablespoons chopped raw almonds
1 tablespoon unsweetened, shredded coconut
¼ teaspoon cinnamon

Combine banana, berries, oats and raisins in a microwave-safe dish. Microwave for 2 minutes. Top with almonds, cinnamon and coconut and microwave for 1 minute. Serve warm.

Men: Double the recipe

LUNCH

JAMAICAN JERK VEGETABLE SALAD
(or leftover Sweet Potato Stew)
2 SERVINGS

¼ teaspoon dried thyme
¼ teaspoon garlic powder
¼ teaspoon dried cinnamon
¼ teaspoon ground allspice
⅛ teaspoon ground black pepper
⅛ teaspoon ground red cayenne pepper
1 cup sliced zucchini
1 small onion, cut into ⅛ inch slices
1 cup sliced red bell pepper
2 Portobello mushrooms, cut into ¼ inch slices
1 teaspoon rice vinegar
2 teaspoons lime juice
⅓ cup black beans
1 mango, peeled and diced, divided
5 ounces mixed baby greens

Combine first six ingredients in a large zip lock plastic bag. Add zucchini, onion, bell pepper, mushrooms, vinegar and lime juice. Seal and shake well to coat.

Lightly wipe a large nonstick skillet with oil. Add vegetable mixture and sauté for 5 minutes or until vegetables are tender, adding a small amount of water if necessary to prevent sticking. Add black beans and ½ cup of the chopped mango and continue cooking for another 2 minutes. Remove from heat.

Serve vegetables on a bed of mixed greens, topped with remaining diced mango.

> **Tip:** A healthful dip or salsa with a variety of colorful raw vegetables is a great way to start a meal. Having a salad or raw vegetables with dip at the beginning of a meal fills you up and prevents overeating.

DINNER

Raw veggies with guacamole, salsa, or hummus
GUACAMOLE
3 SERVINGS

1 medium avocado, peeled and pitted
2 tablespoons diced onions
½ cup roma or plum tomatoes
1 clove fresh garlic, minced
2 teaspoons lime juice
¼ teaspoon ground cumin
2 tablespoons cilantro, chopped

Using a fork, mash the avocado in a medium bowl. Add the remaining ingredients and mix well.

This guacamole should serve 3 people, so share with some friends or if you are dining alone, opt for salsa or hummus.

ZUCCHINI BEAN BURRITO
3 SERVINGS

1 small red onion, chopped
2 cloves garlic, chopped
½ green Poblano chile pepper, seeded and thinly sliced
1 medium tomato chopped
1 small zucchini, chopped
1 ½ cups cooked pinto beans or 1 (15 ounce) can, low sodium or no salt added
½ tablespoon chili powder
½ teaspoon ground cumin
2 tablespoons chopped cilantro
3 large whole grain tortillas
2 cups shredded romaine lettuce or mixed greens
½ cup low sodium salsa
several slices avocado, optional
½ cup cooked shredded chicken, optional

Heat ⅛ cup water in a large skillet. Add onion, garlic and pepper and water sauté until tender, about 3 minutes. Add tomato and zucchini, cover and continue cooking for an additional 5 minutes or until zucchini is soft. Add beans, chili powder, cumin and ¼ cup water, stir to combine and cook for 10 minutes.

Using a potato masher or back of a spoon, thoroughly mash beans. Stir in cilantro and if desired, shredded chicken.

Spread bean mixture on tortillas, top with lettuce, avocado and salsa and roll up.

Gluten-free option: Replace tortillas with lightly-steamed collard leaves

Men: Have 2 burritos

Grapes or other fruit for dessert

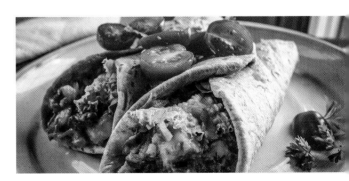

CONGRATULATIONS!
YOU HAVE COMPLETED DAY 20!

Congratulations on completing Day 20 of **10 in 20: Dr. Fuhrman's Lose 10 Pounds in 20 Days Detox Program!** If you have faithfully adhered to the program, you should be feeling healthier, lighter and more energetic than you did 20 days ago. Don't stop now.

If you have met your weight loss goals, you can transition into a healthy maintenance program and make permanent changes to your diet. If you have more weight to lose, you can repeat the menus for one or more additional 20-day cycles or you can begin to design your own menus.

Learn more about my Nutritarian eating style by reading one or more of my books: *Eat to Live* (Little Brown, 2011); *Super Immunity* (HarperOne, 2012); *The End of Diabetes* (HarperOne, 2013); *The Eat to Live Cookbook* (HarperOne, 2013); The End of Dieting (HarperOne, 2014); *The End of Heart Disease* (HarperOne, 2016); *The Eat to Live Quick and Easy Cookbook* (HarperOne, 2017) and *Fast Food Genocide* (HarperOne 2017).

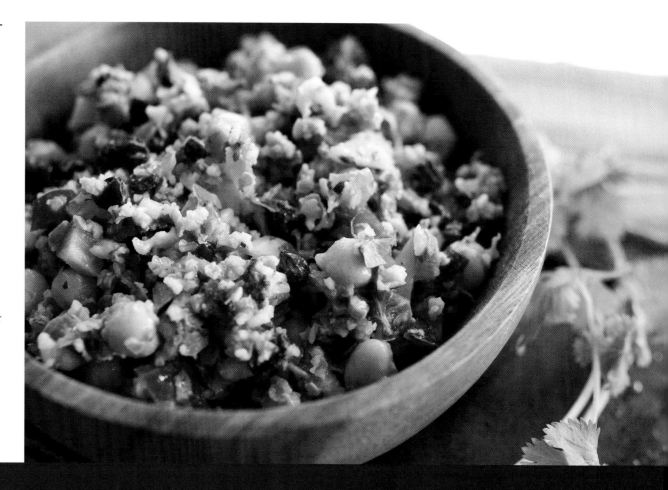

WHAT'S NEXT?

LEARN

Now that you are familiar with how the Nutritarian eating style works, find out more about why it works. The next step on your wellness journey is to read one or more of my *New York Times* best-selling books: *Eat to Live, The End of Dieting, The End of Heart Disease* or *The End of Diabetes*. For parents, there is *Disease-Proof Your Child* and all should read his recent eye-opening work, *Fast Food Genocide*.

These books will give you the in-depth knowledge and practical tools you need to make the Nutritarian eating style your way of life. You'll learn how eating a nutrient-dense, plant-rich diet is a powerful tool for achieving sustainable weight loss and for preventing and reversing chronic diseases, such as heart disease, diabetes, cancer, migraines and autoimmune diseases.
https://shop.drfuhrman.com/books-video

JOIN

Support is a key factor in helping you reach your health and weight loss goals. Membership at DrFuhrman.com gives you that support. You will have access to:

- Nutritarian Recipe database with 1,700+ recipes
- Meal Plans you can download
- Monthly Nutri-Talk / Q&A with Dr. Fuhrman
- Dr. Fuhrman's Video-on-Demand Library

- Position Papers library (download)
- Nutritarian Network online forum
- Living Nutritarian e-magazine (download)
- Connect with Dr. Fuhrman and Dr. Benson in the Ask the Doctor forum**
- Exclusive member promotions

There's a membership level to suit every budget – and you can choose from monthly, annual or lifetime plans.
https://www.drfuhrman.com/membership

* Platinum and Diamond members can post questions in the Ask the Doctor forum. Gold members can view questions and discussions.

GROW

Sometimes, we need extra support when making the transition to the Nutritarian eating style. Dr. Fuhrman's Success Program's licensed clinicians will show you how to put an end to emotional eating, binges, cravings, and other addictive food behaviors. Get the help you need to ensure SUCCESS!

No more addictive food cravings, yo-yo dieting, or emotional eating. Your counselor will:

- Guide you through the foundation of the Nutritarian diet – because knowledge trumps willpower

- Create an action plan based on your unique needs
- Show you how to take action "right now" to make immediate changes in your life
- Review your food diary daily to hold you accountable

Connect with your counselor either in-person at our office, by phone or online – whatever is most convenient for you. Discuss your challenges and gain strategizes for your success! For more information, call our medical practice at (908) 237-0200 or visit
https://www.drfuhrman.com/medical-practice/food-addiction-program

EXPLORE

Support your healthy lifestyle by choosing supplements and food products that are free of problematic ingredients. You can also browse our stock of books, videos and kitchen items. Visit the Shop at DrFuhrman.com for:

- Multivitamins and supplements
- Gourmet foods (soups, dressings, vinegars, Nutrition bars and more)
- *New York Times* best-sellers (print, digital and audio titles)

Also, be sure to check the E-Learning section for updates on Dr. Fuhrman's Guided Detox programs (which take place a few times each year), the Personalized Vitamin Advisor, and the Events section for upcoming U.S. and international vacation getaways with Dr. Fuhrman and his wife, Lisa.

DR. FUHRMAN'S
ADDITIONAL SERVICES

DR. FUHRMAN'S MEDICAL PRACTICE

www.drfuhrman.com/medical-practice
Call for an appointment: (908) 237-0200
Specializing in nutritional and natural medicine to prevent and reverse chronic disease, boost immunity, slow aging and achieve ideal weight and superior health.

In-Office and Remote appointments available.
We offer **Comprehensive medical appointments** (1 hour) and **Condensed medical appointments** (15 minutes). Please note: Condensed medical appointments are scheduled at the sole discretion of the medical office; patients with multiple health issues or complicated diagnoses will be referred to the hour-long comprehensive medical appointment.

Remote consultations available in: California, Florida, Georgia, Illinois, New York, North Carolina, Ohio, Pennsylvania, Texas, Tennessee and Washington

DR. FUHRMAN'S SUCCESS PROGRAM

www.drfuhrman.com/medical-practice/food-addiction-program
Call us today at (908) 237-0200 to find out more.
Put an end to emotional eating, binges, cravings, and other addictive food behaviors with this supportive program.

Our licensed counselor will guide you through the foundation of the Nutritarian diet, create an action plan based on your needs, and review your food diary daily to hold you accountable. Members can take part in a monthly online group chat session.

DR. FUHRMAN'S NUTRITARIAN EDUCATION INSTITUTE

www.drfuhrman.com/nei
Take one course or two and become an expert in the nutrient-dense, plant-rich eating style. Dr. Fuhrman's Nutritarian Studies Program is an online certificate program that teaches the basics of nutrition and the scientific principles behind the Nutritarian eating style. The Art of Nutritarian Cooking certifies you as a Nutritarian chef. The courses are self-paced and structured, with guided lesson plans. * Successful completion of each course may qualify for Continuing Education Unit (CEU) credits.

* Successful completion of each course may qualify for Continuing Education Unit (CEU) credits.

DR. FUHRMAN'S PRODUCTS

https://shop.drfuhrman.com
Browse Dr. Fuhrman's products in the online shop. You'll discover multivitamins for men, women and children; high-quality supplements made from whole-food extracts; food products made without salt, oil, sweeteners or other potentially harmful ingredients; books and media, and much more.

DR. FUHRMAN DESTINATION EVENTS

Enjoy a luxury vacation and health getaway
www.drfuhrman.com/events
Join Dr. Fuhrman and his wife, Lisa, for an unforgettable vacation experience at destinations across the United States and Europe. You'll spend time with Dr. Fuhrman in this relaxed atmosphere, and come back with memories – and important nutritional knowledge – that will last a lifetime. Visit DrFuhrman.com/retreats to view our upcoming events, and make your reservation today.